A WOMAN'S GUIDE TO REGAINING BLADDER CONTROL

NOTE TO READERS:

The authors have provided the material in this book solely for your information. They are not offering any diagnoses or recommending any specific
course of treatment for women with bladder control problems.

In addition, the authors do not have first-hand experience with acupuncture, discussed in Chapter Twelve.

It is essential that you see a physician in order to obtain a proper diagnosis and course of treatment for your individual bladder problem. You should
follow your doctor's instructions carefully, and remain under medical supervision while your condition is being treated.

M. Evans and Company, Inc.
216 East 49th Street
New York, New York 10017

Library of Congress Cataloging-in-Publication Data

Rovner, Eric S.
    A woman's guide to regaining bladder control : everything you need to know
for the diagnosis and cure of incontinence / Eric S. Rovner, Alan J. Wein, and
Donna Caruso.
        p.   cm.
    Includes bibliographical references and index.
    ISBN 0-87131-947-0
    1. Urinary stress incontinence. 2. Bladder—Diseases. 3. Women—Health and
hygiene. I. Wein, Alan J. II. Caruso, Donna. III. Title.
    RG485.S7 R68 2002
    616.6'2—dc21   2002022830

Design and typesetting by Evan Johnston

Printed in the United States of America

9   8   7   6   5   4   3   2   1

A WOMAN'S GUIDE TO REGAINING BLADDER CONTROL

EVERYTHING YOU NEED TO KNOW FOR THE DIAGNOSIS AND CURE OF INCONTINENCE

ERIC S. ROVNER, M.D.
ALAN J. WEIN, M.D.
DONNA CARUSO

M. EVANS AND CO., INC.
NEW YORK

To my wife Michelle, who is incredibly patient, supportive, and beautiful in every way, remaining my lifetime companion and best friend; and to my children, Alexander and Brooke, to whom my only regret in writing this book was the time that I had to spend away from both of you.

—Eric Rovner

To the two most important people in my life, Noele and Nolan, without whose tolerance nothing would get done.

—Alan Wein

To Madeleine Morel, an extraordinary agent, and PJ Dempsey, a remarkable editor.

—Donna Caruso

CONTENTS

PART FOUR: GETTING BETTER

APPENDICES

A WOMAN'S GUIDE TO REGAINING BLADDER CONTROL

INTRODUCTION

If you are one of the millions of women who suffer from the embarrassing and disruptive effects of urinary incontinence—or if you have a close friend or relative who does—this book will bring you new hope.

Sadly, incontinence is one of the great hidden secrets in the women's healthcare field. Despite the greater openness in recent years that has shed light on problems such as male sexual dysfunction, we still rarely hear public discussions about urinary incontinence.

Ranging in severity from the occasional leakage of a few drops of urine to frequent and heavy "accidents," incontinence is a widespread and significant health problem that can be very costly to patients in terms of medical care, medication, and associated products. Clearly, both the general public and the medical profession need to address the problem of incontinence.

So why the silence? There are many reasons, including the following:

- Women are ashamed of the condition and don't want anyone to know they have it.
- Many women falsely believe that incontinence is a natural result of the aging process.
- A large number of people, including some in the healthcare field, mistakenly assume that no effective treatments are available.

As a result, many women go to extremes to hide their condition from family, friends, and coworkers for as long as they can. In some cases, this can go on for many years.

If you are one of these women, you probably know where every bathroom is when you leave your home and you always make sure that one is never more than a few steps away. If there are places where no bathrooms are readily available, you simply don't go there. If the situation gets really bad, you may even give up the job you love because you are constantly running to the bathroom, afraid of humiliating accidents in front of your coworkers.

Perhaps you wear heavy pads and bulky, dark, loose clothing, trying to hide your problem from everyone you know.

Maybe you look for excuses to avoid sex with your partner because you fear urinary leakage during lovemaking.

Or perhaps you refuse to attend important social events such as weddings, birthday parties, or family outings because you are anxious about a possible accident.

As you gradually withdraw more and more from activities you love and from family, friends, and colleagues—who are often baffled by your behavior—the problem just gets worse and worse.

The most unfortunate thing is that you probably do not know how easily you can overcome the problem of incontinence and once again start living your life to the fullest. You just have to learn how to go about it, so let's begin.

Facts You Should Know About Incontinence:

- Urinary incontinence is a very common problem, affecting an estimated fourteen to sixteen million women in this country alone, and probably even more. Some estimates are as high as thirty million women.
- Incontinence is not normal at any age and is not a result of the aging process.
- Incontinence is not a disease, but a symptom of an underlying condition. If you have this problem, it is very important that you seek medical help as soon as possible in order to find out what is wrong and treat it before it gets any worse.
- Incontinence may often be helped by simple, low-cost procedures that do not require surgery, drugs, or lengthy medical treatment.
- Women are up to five times more likely to develop urinary incontinence than men.
- Half the female population will experience urinary incontinence at least once in their lives.
- Only one out of every five women who are affected seeks help for incontinence problems.
- In eighty to ninety percent of cases, treatment can either cure the condition or significantly improve it.
- The real numbers of women with bladder problems may actually be much higher because so many women never report the problem to their doctors to begin with.

How This Book Can Help You

If you experience leakage of urine, there is no reason why you should continue to suffer from this problem. Once you read this book and are aware of all the facts, you will know exactly what to do to get the help you need and deserve.

This book will present the full picture of urinary incontinence in women. It will help you discover the cause of your condition and learn how to go about finding effective care. You will find out what to expect from your medical treatment and how you can use special self-help techniques to improve or even cure your condition.

Along the way, you will also learn about how your urinary system works, how you can figure out if you are really incontinent, and how you can find the best doctor* to treat your condition.

You will find out exactly what information to gather for your doctor and learn what happens in your doctor's office. You will discover how different types of incontinence are diagnosed and why this condition is so often misdiagnosed. You will also find out about some of the medical problems that can cause this condition, including diabetes, infections, and bladder prolapse.

You will learn about the many different treatments that are available and find out about special exercises you can do on your own which may considerably improve your condition.

You will also learn about specific lifestyle changes that can result in significant improvements. For example, you will find out which foods and beverages to avoid because they are often bladder irritants, how smoking can affect incontinence, and why drinking fewer liquids or excessive liquids can actually make your problem worse.

Your feelings won't be overlooked, either. We will help you deal with some of the powerful emotional issues that can affect you as a result of living with this difficult condition, including depression and anxiety.

On a practical level, you will learn about the wide variety of incontinence products that are now available, how they work, and where you can get them. Finally, you will learn how you can find a support group and which organizations you can contact for more information.

In short, this book will be your comprehensive guide to understanding and successfully dealing with the many facets of urinary incontinence and how they affect your life.

As you know, each of us is different, and no one can predict exactly what the results will be once you get the help you need. But this much is certain: you will get better.

---

*NOTE: Although the term "doctor" is generally used in this book, simple and easily managed incontinence can also be treated by other healthcare providers, including physician's assistants, nurse practitioners, and nurse specialists.

How much better? Well, if things go really well, your condition can improve dramatically. You may even be completely cured and no longer have to worry about disrupting your day-to-day life in order to deal with leakage. Many women have experienced complete cures, so let's hope you will be one of them. But even if you aren't, the chances are very high that you will improve considerably with a combination of medical treatment, self-help, and perseverance.

The bottom line is this: If you have any degree of incontinence, there is no need for you to wait any longer. Help is readily available and its effectiveness is beyond question.

So stop worrying about your problem and start doing something about it. Because, as you're about to discover, there's quite a lot you can do to help yourself.

PART I:
WHAT IS INCONTINENCE?

I

WHAT YOU SHOULD KNOW ABOUT INCONTINENCE

THE BASIC FACTS

Like every woman, you are unique and respond to health problems in your own way. On one hand, you may want to know every medical detail of your condition, do extensive research, and ask many questions. On the other hand, you may be content with a knowledge of the basic facts and prefer that your medical choices are closely guided by your doctor. Only you can decide how much you want to know about urinary incontinence, but there are certain facts about this problem that apply to everyone:

Incontinence is the involuntary loss of urine that causes a social or a hygenic problem

- A bladder control problem can develop at any time during your life.
- There are preventive measures that may help to avoid this condition.
- Knowing the facts about incontinence helps in recognizing symptoms in ourselves and in those close to us.
- It is important to seek help immediately.
- People who are well-informed and involved in their treatment usually have a good outcome.

What Is Incontinence and How Does It Affect You?

Here is a simple, comprehensive definition:

Incontinence is the involuntary loss of urine that causes a social or a hygenic problem.

In other words, incontinence is the inability to control your flow of urine. You leak or urinate at times and in places when you don't want to, and this causes you problems socially and hygienically.

Socially, you may be embarrassed because you wet yourself in front of others, whether they are family members, coworkers, or strangers. Your problem makes it difficult to be around other people.

Hygienically, wetting yourself is a problem because you may not be able to change your clothes and clean up right away. As a result, your skin can get raw and red, and you may develop rashes or infections. You may also develop sores, have a bad odor, or other complications.

Even minor incontinence can have a very serious impact on your life.

Who Is Incontinent and Why

You can suffer from this problem at any time during your life. You may be born with it or you can acquire it, perhaps as the result of a urinary tract infection (UTI), surgery, or neurological problems such as multiple sclerosis or spinal cord injuries.

In fact, a very large number of women have—or have had at some time in their lives—a problem controlling their flow of urine. Women are more than twice as likely as men to develop incontinence. Why is it primarily a woman's problem?

Because the structure of the female pelvis and urinary tract makes the female body more prone to the conditions that can result in loss of bladder control. For younger women, pregnancy and childbirth may affect the pelvic muscles and nerves in a way that impairs bladder control. Menopause, resulting in a relatively quick loss of the female hormone estrogen, can be linked to problems with urinary control. For some women, incontinence is only temporary, but for many others, it persists and gets worse over time, especially if it isn't treated.

What Are the Symptoms?

There are several different types of incontinence and they often have different symptoms. The following are typical signs common to all types:

- Loss of urine when performing physical actions such as running, lifting, dancing, laughing, sneezing, or even moving suddenly
- Loss of urine following a sudden and unexpected urge to urinate, leaving no time to get to a bathroom
- Loss of urine accompanied by a feeling that your bladder never empties completely
- Needing to get up many times during the night to urinate and sometimes wetting yourself or the bed
- Needing to urinate more than eight times a day when your liquid intake is normal

When Is Urinary Leakage a Problem?

Do you have a problem you should worry about if you have lost control of your bladder only once? Or if you have a recurring, but very small, dribble from time to time? Or if a little urine comes out during sexual activity?

The only way to discover the underlying cause is through an evaluation by a qualified physician.

The answer is, you can't know for sure. Maybe you do and maybe you don't. The only way to find out is to get a medical evaluation. As urinary leakage can sometimes be a sign of a serious underlying disease, it is always important to discuss it with your doctor as soon as possible. Waiting can result in the underlying condition responsible for causing the incontinence getting much worse, something you definitely want to avoid.

What Causes Incontinence?

It's important to remember that urinary incontinence is not a disease, but rather a *symptom* or an indication of an underlying condition. Some of these conditions may be minor or temporary, but others can be quite serious and require immediate treatment. You will learn the details about all the different possible causes in Chapter Three.

If you are leaking urine, there is a reason this is happening and it is up to you to find out why. Guessing what it might be, or worse yet, not thinking about it, will not help you at all and may even be harmful to your overall health. The only way to discover the underlying cause is through an evaluation by a qualified physician.

Some of the factors that may cause or aggravate bladder control problems include:

- Weakness of the pelvic floor muscles
- Lowered estrogen levels, especially after menopause
- Urinary tract infections

- Pelvic injuries
- Diabetes
- Obesity
- Chronic coughing, as with asthma, bronchitis, or smoking
- Multiple sclerosis
- Parkinson's disease
- Stroke
- Spinal cord injuries
- Radiation therapy
- Pelvic surgery, including hysterectomy, rectal operations, and previous surgery for incontinence
- Back injury or back surgery
- Bladder, uterine, or other pelvic organ prolapse (the organ moves out of its proper place)
- Chronic constipation
- Pregnancy
- Childbirth
- Depression
- Dementia
- Genetic factors
- Certain medications
- Alcohol
- Caffeine
- Certain foods

You may think you know the cause of your incontinence, or you may be convinced that it will go away, especially if it occurs after you have a baby and learn that friends and relatives had the same problem for a short time.

But you may be wrong. That's why it is always best to discuss any urinary leakage with your doctor and find out exactly what is going on.

Don't be afraid because the cause of incontinence is *not* a serious underlying disease for most women and can be cured or treated, as you will see in Chapter 3.

Before we get to that, let's go over exactly how a woman's urinary system is designed to work.

2

HOW A WOMAN'S URINARY SYSTEM WORKS

In order to understand why your urinary system (or urinary tract) isn't working properly, it's important to understand how it is designed and how it works when everything is normal.

Most of the female urinary system is found in the pelvis, the bowl-shaped area between your waist and your thighs. The urinary system has two main purposes: storing urine and eliminating urine (in a way that you are able to control).

When you are continent and everything is working properly, your body holds the urine in your bladder until you are ready to empty it through urinating (also called *micturition* or voiding).

THE PARTS OF THE URINARY SYSTEM

The urinary system consists of:

- *The kidneys* are two organs that remove waste products from the blood and create urine, then send the urine through the ureters to the bladder. On average, the kidneys produce between one and a half and two quarts of urine daily
- *The ureters* are two thin, muscular tubes that carry urine from the kidneys to the bladder
- *The bladder* is a muscular sack, shaped like a balloon and located in the pelvic cavity, that holds urine
- *The urethra* is a hollow tube or canal that carries urine from the bladder out of the body.

Muscles Involved in Urination

Although they are not considered part of the urinary system, the following three types of muscles play important parts in the urinary process:

- *The urethral sphincter muscles* are located in the wall of the urethra. This band of muscles tightly holds the urethra closed, thereby preventing the loss of urine from the bladder. When these muscles relax, they open, allowing urine to pass out of the bladder and then out of the body.

- *The pelvic floor muscles* are shaped like a sling at the bottom of the pelvic bowl. These muscles act to support the bladder, uterus, and rectum and keep them in place. They also help keep the urethra closed so no urine leaks out.

- *The detrusor muscle* is the muscle responsible for squeezing the urine out of the bladder through the urethra during urination.

Steps in the Urinary Process

After you eat and drink, your body digests this food for the body to use as fuel. The unusable parts of your food are discarded as solid and liquid waste. The liquid waste is sent through the bloodstream to the kidneys, where it is filtered and turned into urine. The urine is then conducted down the ureters and into the bladder, where it is stored. This process continues every minute of every day in a healthy person.

When the bladder is almost full of urine (the average bladder holds eight to twelve ounces of urine), the nerves in the bladder send a message to the brain which results
in that familiar urge which lets you know that you have to urinate.

When you sit down to urinate, the pelvic floor muscles, which have been holding in the urine, relax. The urethral sphincter muscles also relax, opening the urethra. At the same time, the muscles in your bladder contract, squeezing the stored urine out and allowing it to pass through the urethra and out of the body.

Finally, when the urination process is complete and the bladder is empty, the bladder muscles stop squeezing and relax again. The sphincter and pelvic floor muscles tighten to hold in the new supply of urine that will be entering the bladder as the process continues.

Holding It In

When the body works normally, it is possible to resist the urge to urinate and "hold it in," even for as long as many hours. The healthy body is designed to delay urination when needed. If you can't get to the toilet, the brain sends a signal that the body is not ready to release the urine, which causes the pelvic floor muscles to remain taut, holding the urethra closed so no urine can escape. Holding these muscles taut also sends a signal back to the detrusor muscle of your bladder, which suppresses or prevents this muscle from squeezing the urine into the urethra.

As you will see, when complications arise, things don't always work so smoothly.

3

THE MANY CAUSES OF INCONTINENCE

You Need Help No Matter What the Cause

There are many causes for urinary incontinence, ranging from very minor conditions that often cure themselves to serious medical conditions requiring long-term treatment.

No matter how insignificant your urinary leakage, if you have this problem, you must seek immediate help. The reason is that you don't know what may be causing your incontinence until it is diagnosed and the cause could be something that requires treatment.

Physical Conditions That Can Cause Incontinence

Many physical conditions can cause incontinence, including the following:

Pregnancy

Pregnant women experience the need to urinate often, accompanied by periodic urinary incontinence. The most likely cause is the additional weight and pressure of the growing baby, which is pressing down on the pelvic area, especially on the bladder, but also on the urethra and pelvic floor muscles.

This additional pressure reduces the size and capacity of the bladder, so it can't hold its usual amount of urine. As a result, when you are pregnant, you have to urinate far more often than usual.

Loss of bladder control during pregnancy can result from weakness in the pelvic floor muscles. These weakened muscles are not as able to hold in the urine completely, so some of it leaks out.

During pregnancy, it is always important for your doctor to be aware of any sign of incontinence because certain causes, such as urinary tract infections, need to be treated.

However, most instances of urinary frequency and incontinence are normal byproducts of pregnancy and require no treatment. They usually go away by themselves shortly after the child is born but it is best to be sure and alert your doctor to any sign of urinary leakage.

Childbirth

Giving birth (especially vaginally) puts additional pressure and weight on the pelvic area. During childbirth, the baby pushes on the bladder, urethra, and pelvic muscles, which can weaken the sphincter and pelvic floor muscles, making it more likely that these muscles will not be strong enough to prevent urinary leakage.

As the pelvic floor muscles are forced to stretch out as the baby emerges, they can be weakened and lead to urinary incontinence, sometimes shortly after childbirth and sometimes many years later.

In addition, pregnancy and childbirth may have other damaging effects on the urinary system:

- The bladder and urethra can be moved out of their proper positions.
- The nerves that control the bladder and urethra may be damaged.
- An episiotomy can damage and weaken the pelvic floor muscles.

Menopause and the Decline of Hormones

The female hormone estrogen is also essential in maintaining a healthy urinary system, although this association has not been definitely proven scientifically. During menopause, estrogen levels drop, which may be associated with problems linked to urinary incontinence.

Lower estrogen levels result in changes in the urinary tract tissues, making them less elastic and more rigid. As a result, urinary incontinence may occur. In addition, infections, such as cystitis, which are linked to incontinence, may also occur with more frequency following menopause.

Sometimes this problem is treated by prescribing supplemental estrogen, either as a cream, a patch, or an oral medication. In many cases, the application of a topical estrogen-containing cream to the urethra and vagina may be sufficient to alleviate the condition.

The Aging Process

While incontinence is not a natural result of the aging process, changes in older bodies can definitely make the problem worse. As we age, our muscles tend to lose some of their strength and elasticity. They become stiff and unable to expand easily, and the pelvic muscles may not be able to hold in urine as well as in the past.

A woman who has given birth to a few children may also have weakened sphincter and pelvic floor muscles, or pelvic organ prolapse. This, combined with loss of estrogen and the consequent changes in body tissues can cause further problems. In some women, there may also be damage from a neurological disease, such as a stroke, Parkinson's disease, or Alzheimer's disease. In such cases, the message to urinate from body to brain simply doesn't get through or is delayed.

The point is that for most of us, getting older does not necessarily mean that urinary incontinence is inevitable. There are many things we can do to prevent the condition or, if it is already present, to improve or cure it.

Obesity

Fat deposits put additional pressure on the pelvis, particularly the pelvic floor muscles, in women who are overweight (ten to twenty percent over the ideal weight). Depending on the degree of obesity and how long a woman remains obese, these muscles can weaken over time, leading to urinary leakage.

This means that if you have bladder control problems and are also overweight, one of your first steps toward controlling incontinence is to lose the excess weight, then, continue on a program to keep it off.

INFECTIONS AND MEDICAL DISORDERS

The following physical disorders and diseases can result in urinary incontinence. If you have, or suspect you have any of these, you should consult your physician.

Urinary Tract Infections

Urinary tract infections (UTIs) are common bacterial infections in any part of the urinary system, including the bladder, kidneys, ureters, or urethra. The infection causes an irritation of the lining of the bladder, making it less able to contain urine. During the course of a UTI, the bladder may become irritable and spastic and contract involuntarily. The urine then begins to leak out, resulting in periodic incontinence.

How do the bacteria get inside the body and create these infections? Normally, there are no infectious bacteria present in the bladder, but there are infectious bacteria that thrive outside the body on the skin, in the vagina, and also in the rectum and in stool. It is the bacteria that live in and around the vagina that most often gain entry into the bladder to cause infections.

One method of preventing UTIs is to always wipe yourself front to back following a bowel movement. This method will keep rectal bacteria from travelling into the vagina and up to the bladder, infecting it.

Most urinary tract infections are easily cured with the use of antibiotics. If you have any symptoms of this problem, get help right away before it develops into something far worse.

Cystitis

Although many women use the terms "cystitis" and "urinary tract infection" interchangeably, they are not really the same thing. Cystitis, an inflammation of the urinary bladder, is one type of UTI that can result from bacteria entering the bladder. Another type of UTI is a kidney infection; this is also known as pyelonephritis. If you are healthy, your body is usually able to fight off and destroy bacteria. Sometimes, either because there are large numbers or especially virulent bacteria, or because part your immune system is weakened, an infection takes hold. Then, the bacteria begin to grow and multiply, causing the bladder to become painful and inflamed.

The symptoms of cystitis include:

- Bladder pain, which is sometimes alleviated after urination
- Burning or stinging during urination (called *dysuria*)
- A feeling of fullness in the bladder, even when it is not full
- A need to urinate very often
- Discolored urine (darker or cloudier than normal)
- A sudden urgency to urinate
- Uncontrollable urinary leakage
- Frequent waking at night to urinate
- General fatigue

"Honeymoon cystitis" is a common condition that results from repeated sexual activity that can push bacteria from the vagina into the urethra and bladder, causing infection. Studies have also shown that women who use a diaphragm for contraception are more likely to develop cystitis because the diaphragm can bring in bacteria if it is not totally clean when inserted. In addition, spermicide seems to compound the problem, since it encourages bacterial growth inside the vagina.

It is very important to report any sudden urinary tract distress to your doctor. If a urinary tract infection is not treated right away, the infection may spread to the kidneys, where serious damage can occur. A bacterial infection of the kidneys causes chills, high fever, and back pain, and requires immediate treatment. Otherwise, it can continue to spread, possibly to your blood, where it can eventually cause serious illness or even death if it's not treated right away.

Interstitial Cystitis

The symptoms for interstitial cystitis are very similar to those of urinary tract infections and it is easy to confuse one with the other. But there is a significant difference: interstitial cystitis is not definitely caused by bacteria. In fact, the cause (or causes) of this condition remains unknown.

Interstitial cystitis predominantly affects women, causing severe urinary symptoms, including pelvic, vaginal, urethral or bladder pain, and strong feelings of urinary urgency. It also results in a feeling that your bladder will burst if you don't get to the bathroom immediately, but then, when you urinate, only a small amount comes out. Only very rarely does interstitial cystitis cause incontinence.

At times, interstitial cystitis can be so severe that it causes causes permanent scarring on the bladder wall, resulting in decreasing the size of the bladder. In fact, in some cases, the bladder may only be able to hold one or two ounces of liquid, as opposed to the normal eight to twelve ounces.

The symptoms of interstitial cystitis include:

- Pain in the bladder, urethra, vaginal, or pelvic area
- A feeling of pressure in these areas
- A strong sense of urgency, or needing to get to the bathroom quickly

• A frequent need to urinate, as often as once every half hour or even more, around the clock
• Pain during sexual intercourse

If you experience any of these symptoms, you should report them to your doctor immediately.

There are several ways to treat interstitial cystitis, but there is no cure at this time. You may be given medication or may find relief through the elimination of certain foods from your diet (see Chapter Eleven).

The symptoms of interstitial cystitis can be weak or strong and they can also fluctuate, with some days quite painful and others far more comfortable. These symptoms can be very similar to those of urinary tract infections, which is one reason why a prompt and proper diagnosis is so essential.

Pelvic Organ Prolapse

Pelvic organ prolapse occurs when one of the organs located in the pelvis, such as the bladder, moves out of place. The primary reason this happens is because the organ loses its support and falls or pushes into the vagina, usually due to weakening of the pelvic floor muscles that hold the organs in place.

A prolapsed bladder that sags into the vagina is called a *cystocele.* When the bladder is not in its proper place, this can result in bladder overactivity, urinary obstruction, and/or stress incontinence. Other pelvic organs, such as the uterus, may also move out of place, creating problems for the normal urinary process.

There are many things can trigger a pelvic organ prolapse, including:

• Vaginal childbirth
• Loss of estrogen following menopause
• Obesity
• Chronic coughing (as with asthma, bronchitis, or smoking)
• Heavy lifting
• Continual straining (as with constipation)

Pelvic organ prolapse may be classified in three ways: mild, moderate, or severe, and can result in urinary incontinence. Other types of pelvic organ prolapse include rectal prolapse (*rectocele*), intestinal prolapse (*enterocele*) and prolapse of the uterus. Some of the symptoms of prolapse include:

- Pain or pressure in the lower back
- Difficulty urinating or defecating
- An uncomfortable feeling that a lump is protruding from the vagina
- Pain or discomfort during sexual intercourse

Treatment for pelvic organ prolapse includes supportive devices (see Chapter Fifteen), Kegel exercises (see Chapter Eleven), and in some cases, surgery (see chapter Fourteen.)

Neurological Disorders

When the urinary process works properly, pelvic nerves send a message via the spinal cord and to the brain that the bladder is full and needs to be emptied. The brain then sends a signal that it's time to head for the bathroom, followed by the message to the nerves to empty the bladder.

If nerves are damaged, this process doesn't always work properly. The message may never get through to the spinal cord or brain, or the brain may be unable to get the message back to the body. The result is that either the brain or the body, or both, never get the message that you have to urinate and urine flows unexpectedly.

There are many conditions that can cause the nerve damage that results in urinary incontinence, including:

- Diabetes (see below)
- Spinal cord injuries
- Stroke
- Alzheimer's disease
- Multiple sclerosis
- Parkinson's disease
- Back injury or surgery

- Poliomyelitis
- Dementia
- Spina bifida and other congenital disorders

When nerves are damaged, other things can occur. There may be problems with the nerves responsible for storage of urine in the bladder, resulting in urinary leakage. Or there may be problems that do not allow the bladder to empty completely, which result in urine leakage, even after urination.

These neurological disorders don't always cause incontinence, and that's one reason why a physician needs to make a diagnosis. If one of these conditions is the cause of your bladder control problem, it can often be successfully treated with measures such as behavioral modification (see Chapter Eleven), medication (see Chapter Thirteen), or rarely, surgery (see Chapter Fourteen).

Diabetes

The neurological changes diabetes brings about can often create urinary incontinence. In fact, involuntary loss of urine is a common side effect of this disorder.

Diabetes can cause damage to the nerves involved with the urinary process, especially those associated with the bladder. This means that the message that the bladder is full may never reach the spinal cord or the brain, causing the bladder to continue to fill and finally overflow, causing leakage, since the brain isn't aware that the bladder needs to be emptied.

A common symptom of untreated diabetes is excessive thirst. People with undiagnosed and untreated diabetes tend to consume a lot of fluids and therefore need to urinate more often than usual. Since diabetes also damages muscles and/or nerves, it is possible that a person suffering from this disease may not be able to control urination, so leakage occurs.

Today, diabetes is a treatable disease and many people live long and productive lives once they learn how to keep their blood sugar under control. Be sure to see your doctor if you think you might have diabetes. Early detection can prevent permanent damage to the bladder and other internal organs. If not treated, diabetes can be fatal.

PELVIC SURGERY

Sometimes, incontinence can result from pelvic surgery. In women, hysterectomy is the most common type of pelvic surgery. In fact, approximately 600,000 hysterectomies are performed each year in the United States alone.

A recent study shows that women who have had hysterectomies have a much higher risk of developing urinary incontinence than women who have not had this surgery. Specifically, the study found that women who have undergone hysterectomies have a 60 percent greater risk of incontinence by the time they reach the age of sixty. In many cases, the condition doesn't develop until many years after the surgery. The researchers said that the reasons for this finding are still uncertain.

What this means is that if you develop bladder problems following hysterectomy, a diagnostic evaluation, including urodynamics (see chapter Nine), may determine whether the surgery is related to the incontinence and also what type of incontinence you have developed.

Incontinence may also develop following other types of pelvic surgery, including caesarean sections, rectal operations, surgery for pelvic cancers or vaginal prolapse, and radical colon operations. Even surgery for incontinence itself can occasionally lead to a worsening of the condition.

The reason is that pelvic surgery can cause damage to the pelvic nerves and muscles, and sometimes even to the bladder. Although this doesn't happen too often, it is still a good idea for you to consider it as a possible cause when discussing your condition with your physician, so don't forget to inform your doctor about any pelvic surgery you may have had.

Medications

One of the most frequently overlooked causes of urinary incontinence is medication. Many prescription or over-the-counter drugs have side effects that can contribute to loss of bladder control.

When this is the case, it is one of the easiest types of incontinence to correct. When you talk to your doctor about your bladder control problem, remember to bring a list of all prescription and over-the-counter medications you are taking (see Chapter Eight.)

Some of the prescription medications that are associated with bladder control problems are:

- Sedatives, such as diazepam (Valium)
- Muscle relaxants, such as chlordiazepoxide (Librium)
- Diuretics, such as furosemide (Lasix)
- Anticholinergics, such as propantheline bromide (Pro-Banthine)
- Calcium channel blockers, such as diltiazem (Cardizem)
- Antidepressants/antipsychotics, such as amitriptyline (Elavil) or haloperidol (Haldol)
- Narcotics, such as meperidine (Demerol)
- Antihypertensives, such as doxazosin (Cardura) or terazosin (Hytrin)

Some of the over-the-counter medications that can cause bladder control problems include:

- Antihistamines with diphenhydramine (Benadryl)
- Sedatives with diphenhydramine (Excedrin P.M.)
- Stimulants with caffeine (No Doz)
- Analgesics with diphenhydramine (Tylenol PM)
- Cough medications with pseudoephedrine (Robitussin)
- Diet pills with phenylpropanolamine (Dexatrim)

You should also check the package insert on any drugs you now take to see if urinary problems are listed among the possible side effects. If you don't have a package insert, ask your pharmacist, consult a drug guide, or ask the doctor who has prescribed the drug.

If you suspect your problem has resulted from taking a non-prescription, over-the-counter medication, consider stopping it. Consult the package insert and then call your doctor to see if there is an alternative medication. If there is one ingredient in a medication (prescription or non-prescription) that is causing incontinence, your doctor can almost always prescribe another, similar medication that will not give you the same unwanted side effect.

It is really important for you to remember not to self-diagnose and act as your own doctor. *Never stop taking a prescription medication without instructions from your doctor.* If you think it may be causing a bladder control problem, contact your physician first.

DIETARY FACTORS

Sometimes, incontinence can be caused or made worse by things you eat or drink. Certain substances are irritants to the bladder and may make it harder to control the urinary process. They include:

Never stop taking a prescription medication without instructions from your doctor

- Caffeine (coffee, tea, soft drinks)
- Alcohol
- Carbonated beverages (with or without caffeine)
- Milk and milk products
- Citrus juice and citrus fruits
- Tomatoes and tomato products
- Chocolate
- Sweeteners (sugar, honey, corn syrup)
- Artificial sweeteners (aspartame, saccharin)
- Spicy foods

In most cases, these foods do not cause incontinence all by themselves; and they appear to aggravate problems that already exist in some cases. The exact reasons why these substances may contribute to incontinence are not yet known.

If you think that any of the above food items may be causing you a problem, it is a good idea to eliminate some or all of them from your diet and see if your bladder condition improves. If it does, you can try re-introducing them one at a time, as a way to pinpoint the culprit(s). It's a good idea to have your doctor monitor this approach.

OTHER POSSIBLE CAUSES OF URINARY INCONTINENCE

You can see from the following exhaustive list, urinary incontinence can have many different causes. Even if you think you might know what is causing your condition, you may not be wrong or you may be only partially wrong.

• Family history of incontinence
• Birth defects, such as spina bifida
• Pelvic injuries
• Dementia
• Radiation therapy in the pelvic area
• Chronic cough, as from asthma, bronchitis, or smoking
• Chronic straining, as with constipation
• Uterine fibroids
• Fistula (a hole in the bladder)
• Certain types of cancers, including those of the bladder

IT MAY NOT BE URINE

Do not automatically assume that you have a bladder control problem if you find that your underpants are wet.

The only way to find out whether or not you are really leaking urine is to have a doctor examine you. Sometimes vaginal secretions can be copious enough to appear as urine. These may be entirely normal or could also be a symptom of another medical problem. Again, this is something you can't really determine on your own and need to have checked out with your doctor. The bottom line is that you should see your doctor if you experience any type of wetness that you cannot control.

4

THE FIVE TYPES OF INCONTINENCE

There are five main types of incontinence: stress urinary incontinence (SUI), urge incontinence (which includes reflex incontinence), mixed incontinence, overflow incontinence, and total incontinence. It is possible for you to suffer from only one type or from a combination of different types. It is essential that you receive an accurate diagnosis, so the appropriate treatment can be prescribed to treat your specific condition. With proper treatment, you have up to a 90 percent chance of finding either a complete cure or significant help.

STRESS URINARY INCONTINENCE (SUI)

SUI is the most common type of incontinence. Although with SUI, sometimes only small amounts of urine come out, that is often enough to cause embarrassment and other personal problems.

It is important to realize that the "stress" in stress incontinence does not mean anxiety. SUI (*exertional* incontinence might be a better name) occurs when additional pressure or stress is put on the bladder. This condition affects women of all ages, but the condition is more common in older women. Its main cause is weakened sphincter or pelvic floor muscles that are not able to completely hold in urine when pressure is applied to the abdomen and bladder through sneezing, coughing, straining, exercising, or lifting. In really severe cases, leakage can occur from something as simple as getting up from a chair or walking normally.

As you have seen in Chapter Two, the pelvic floor muscles hold up the bladder and assist in keeping the urethra closed until urination occurs. When these muscles lose their normal strength, it causes the bladder neck and urethra to "drop" in some women. Then, when additional pressure is applied, some urine is able to leak out because the sphincter muscles can't compensate and keep the (or prolapsed) bladder neck and urethra closed. Other women with stress incontinence may not have a "dropped" bladder, but nonetheless have leakage due to intrinsic weakness of the urethral sphincter muscles alone.

SUI is most common in women who have given birth vaginally, because the pelvic floor muscles and nerves stretch during delivery. It has been estimated that up to 30 percent of women experience some stress incontinence for six to twelve months after giving birth. Usually, the incontinence goes away by itself, but that is not always the case, and the assistance of your doctor may be needed.

Stress incontinence caused by childbirth may not appear until many years later, since weakened muscles may get worse over time. This is especially true in women who have given birth to several children.

If you experience episodes of stress incontinence, it does not necessarily occur only when you have a full bladder. This means that you may not have a feeling that you need to urinate when the incontinence happens. In fact, with this type of incontinence, leakage can occur when there is only a small amount of urine in the bladder. You become aware of the problem only when you discover that you are wet.

The Major Symptoms of Stress Incontinence

- Urine loss during coughing, sneezing, sudden movements, exercise, laughing, or lifting
- No urine loss during sleep
- Sudden spurts of urine loss *not* associated with a sense of urgency

Associations or Causes of Stress Incontinence

- Loss of estrogen after menopause
- Pelvic surgery, such as hysterectomy, rectal operations, and previous surgery for incontinence
- Pelvic organ prolapse (bladder, uterus, or rectum)
- Obesity
- Chronic cough, from asthma, bronchitis, or smoking
- Changes due to aging, such as weakened sphincter muscle or impaired nerve function
- Effects of other disorders including diabetes, stroke, and pelvic tumors
- Childbirth

Urge Incontinence

Urge incontinence is characterized by repeated instances of strong, sudden urges to urinate that leave no time to get to the bathroom. If you find yourself running to the bathroom and not always getting there in time, you are suffering from urge incontinence. With urge incontinence, urine passes uncontrollably in large amounts—sometimes it may even be the entire contents of the bladder.

This type of incontinence, which can vary in its severity, is more likely to develop as you grow older. The most common cause is irritability and involuntary contractions or spasm of the detrusor muscle of the bladder wall (see Chapter Two). These contractions result in a sudden rise in pressure within the bladder and the forced expulsion of urine out through the urethra.

The term *overactive bladder* describes the condition resulting from multiple involuntary bladder contractions. The symptoms of overactive bladder include urinary frequency, urgency, waking up at night to urinate, and urge urinary incontinence. An overactive bladder may be the cause of urge incontinence, but not every woman with an overactive bladder leaks urine. In fact, of the estimated fourteen to sixteen million women suffering from bladder overactivity, only about a third have urge incontinence. The others, who need to urinate frequently, are able to get to the bathroom in time.

One of the worst things about urge incontinence is that it can happen at any time—even immediately after urination—day or night. In some cases, it can be set off by drinking a small amount of liquid or even by just hearing the sound of running water.

The Major Symptoms of Urge Incontinence

- A strong, uncontrollable need to urinate and a frequent inability to get to the toilet in time
- Leakage of large amounts of urine
- Frequent urination, especially more than eight times a day and not always making it to the toilet in time
- Wetting the bed or having to get up frequently at night to urinate and not always reaching the toilet in time

Associated Conditions

- Urinary tract infections (cystitis)
- Neurological disorders such as stroke, spinal cord injuries, Parkinson's disease, Alzheimer's disease, or multiple sclerosis
- Urinary tract obstruction
- Pelvic surgery, such as radical pelvic surgery for cancer
- Radiation therapy
- Chronic constipation

• Anxiety disorders
• Diabetes

REFLEX INCONTINENCE

Reflex incontinence may be considered another type of urge incontinence in which there is a loss of urine due to an involuntary bladder contraction, but without any warning or sensation of urgency.

Why? Because the nerves have been damaged, perhaps by medical conditions that leave them unable to carry the message that you need to urinate to your brain. Since there is no sensation of the need to void, urination happens suddenly, unpredictably, and without any awareness.

CAUSES OF REFLEX INCONTINENCE

• Neurological disorders, such as spinal cord injuries
• Pelvic surgery, such as radical pelvic surgery for cancer
• Radiation therapy

In general, you can think of all types of urge incontinence as having a bladder that misbehaves. If the bladder contracts and releases urine without your conscious permission and without giving you enough time to get to the bathroom to avoid an accident, you are probably suffering from urge incontinence and you should see your doctor (see Chapter Nine).

Mixed Incontinence

If you have read the descriptions of stress incontinence and urge incontinence and are confused about which type you have, or discover that you experience some of the symptoms of both types, you may be suffering from what is called mixed incontinence. This condition is quite common and, as the name implies, results from a combination of both stress and urge incontinence.

If you have mixed incontinence, the symptoms of either stress or urge incontinence are usually stronger or more troublesome. Figuring out which type is predominant is essential in helping to determine the best course of treatment.

Of all the types of incontinence, stress, urge and mixed account for an estimated ninety percent of all cases of incontinence.

OVERFLOW INCONTINENCE

This form of the incontinence requires immediate attention because you can become very ill with serious conditions such as kidney damage or urinary tract infections that can lead to blood poisoning

Overflow incontinence, which is far less common than the three types already discussed, occurs when the bladder does not empty completely or when the body produces more urine than the bladder can hold and it becomes overfilled. The result is a spill-over effect, and an involuntary leakage of urine.

It is important to realize that with overflow incontinence, the bladder is never able to empty completely. When you have overflow incontinence, the bladder is always full. Even when you think you have emptied the bladder, and you feel like the bladder is empty, it isn't. That is the central problem.

Not everyone with overflow incontinence has the feeling that the bladder is full, but they all experience some loss of urine, which can happen at any time, day or night. It happens because the bladder is full or is never emptied completely, and therefore urine leaks out when more is produced.

Overflow incontinence is more common in men than in women because it is often a result of a blockage that prevents the bladder from emptying completely. In men, this frequently results from an enlarged prostate gland which impinges on the urethra, causing blockage of urine as it exits the bladder. In women, it most commonly happens from a neurological condition, such as multiple sclerosis or diabetes.

If you suffer from this type of incontinence, you must get medical treatment. This form of the incontinence requires immediate attention because you can become very ill with serious conditions such as kidney damage or urinary tract infections that can lead to blood poisoning (sepsis).

Causes of Overflow Incontinence

1. One cause is weakness of the bladder's detrusor muscle (see chapter 2), as a result of problems including:
   - Diabetes
   - Multiple sclerosis
   - Pelvic surgery, such as radical pelvic surgery for cancer
   - Pelvic injuries
   - Pelvic organ prolapse
   - Disc problems in the spine
   - Alcoholism
   - Shingles (herpes zoster)
   - Polio
   - Long-term practice of holding urine in for hours at a time, causing overdistention and overstretching of the detrusor muscle

2. Another cause may be obstructions in or near the bladder caused by:
   - Stricture or narrowing of the urethra
   - Constriction or overgrowth of the bladder neck muscle
   - Neurological disease, such as spinal cord injury or multiple sclerosis
   - Prior bladder surgery

Symptoms of Overflow Incontinence

- Leakage of small amounts of urine during both the day and the night
- An urge to urinate, but nothing comes out
- The feeling of having a full or partly full bladder, but only being able to urinate a small amount
- The need to urinate frequently during the night

- Spending a lot of time trying to urinate and either not succeeding or only voiding a small amount
- A constant uncontrollable dribbling of urine throughout the day and night
- Weak force of stream

Total Incontinence

Total incontinence means not having any control of the bladder. A person with total incontinence does not know when the bladder is full or partly full and is not even aware of the need to empty it.

The usual cause of total incontinence is nerve damage to the nervous system, which interferes with the body's ability to signal the brain and the relevant organs that there is a need to use the toilet. This nerve damage can have many causes, including:

- Dementia
- Spinal cord injuries
- Pelv ic surgery for cancer

If you have been diagnosed with total incontinence as a result of nerve damage, you should remain under your doctor's care. This condition usually requires ongoing medical supervision.

OTHER TYPES OF INCONTINENCE

There are several other types of incontinence that are rare in comparison to the major types of incontinence already discussed, but it is important to know about them so that you can consider every possibility when making a diagnosis. Some of the other kinds of incontinence include the following.

Incontinence Due to Surgery

Sometimes surgical procedures can result in urinary incontinence. Hysterectomy, caesarean section for childbirth, or surgery of the rectum or lower intestinal tract may result in a fistula if the bladder is nicked during surgery. A fistula is an abnormal connection (a hole) between your bladder and vagina which results in the continuous leakage of urine into your vagina. Fistulas may also occur from some types of cancers and they almost never go away by themselves.

Transient Incontinence

This type of incontinence is temporary and reversible with proper medical treatment. Causes include urinary tract infections, vaginitis, and some medications, including diuretics. It can also be caused by vaginal childbirth; in that case, it often goes away by itself within six months to a year.

Congenital Incontinence:

During fetal development, certain malformations may occur in the development of the urinary tract, resulting in a urinary system that does not work properly because it is not formed normally. Although this is a rare cause for urinary leakage, it does occur and individuals are treated on a case-by-case basis, depending upon what type of malformation needs to be corrected. People with congenital incontinence have lived with this problem since birth.

5

HOW TO DETERMINE IF YOU ARE INCONTINENT

THE ESSENTIAL FACTS ABOUT INCONTINENCE

By now, you should be aware of two very important facts:

- If you have an involuntary loss of urine, which means urine that leaks out when you don't want it to, you are incontinent.

• If you are incontinent, you should see your doctor right away.

Even when you are aware of these facts, you may still be confused about whether or not you have a medical problem that requires treatment. The incontinence questionnaire below may help to clarify the situation.

Scoring the Questionnaire

Answering the following questions may be helpful in determining whether you have a bladder control problem and, if so, how extensive it is and what the possible cause or causes may be. The answers can also be very useful if you bring the information to your doctor on your first visit (see chapter 8).

The truth is that you don't really need this quiz to decide whether or not you need medical assistance. If you have any urinary leakage at all, even if it is only a small amount and even if it only happened once, there is a possibility that you may have significant incontinence.

If you suspect incontinence, it is important for you to have it diagnosed and treated immediately, before the underlying condition that is causing it gets any worse. Many medical conditions develop quite rapidly and a delay in treatment can be crucial to your health.

In many other cases, the situation is only temporary and goes away by itself, or can be treated with changes in medication or diet, or by the simple exercises you will learn about in Chapter Eleven.

The odds are very much in your favor that a simple cause will be found for your incontinence and that a painless, non-invasive treatment will either cure it or dramatically improve it. What's important is that you overcome any reluctance you may feel and seek help as soon as possible.

Risk Factors

If you have had an incontinence problem, your lifestyle, medical history, or heredity may be contributing to it. The following is a list of the risk factors for incontinence. If you answer "yes" to any of these questions, it's possible that this specific risk factor is a contributor to your type of incontinence..

INCONTINENCE QUESTIONNAIRE

1. Are you a smoker?   *Yes* ❏   *No* ❏

2. Are you overweight (ten to twenty percent over the ideal weight for your height and age)   *Yes* ❏   *No* ❏

3. Are you an excessive drinker of alcohol?   *Yes* ❏   *No* ❏

4. Have you gone through menopause?   *Yes* ❏   *No* ❏

5. Have you had pelvic surgery?   *Yes* ❏   *No* ❏

6. Are you diabetic, or do you have any of the other medical conditions mentioned in chapter 3 that can be associated with incontinence (UTIs, cystitis, interstitial cystitis, pelvic organ prolapse, neurological disorders including spinal cord injuries, stroke, Alzheimer's disease, multiple sclerosis, Parkinson's disease, back injury or back surgery, poliomyelitis, dementia, spina bifida)?   *Yes* ❏   *No* ❏

7. Do you have a problem with constipation and straining in the bathroom?   *Yes* ❑   *No* ❑

8. Have you ever given birth vaginally?   *Yes* ❑   *No* ❑

9. Have you ever been treated for urinary tract infections, including cystitis?   *Yes* ❑   *No* ❑

10. Does your urinary leakage seem worse when you eat certain foods or drink certain beverages?   *Yes* ❑   *No* ❑

11. Are you on any medications that have incontinence as a possible side effect?   *Yes* ❑   *No* ❑

12. Has anyone in your family, especially your parents or siblings, suffered from incontinence?   *Yes* ❑   *No* ❑

SYMPTOMS

Each of the following symptoms is related to a form of incontinence. If you have any of them, see your doctor for a complete diagnosis and treatment plan.

13. Do you have pain when you urinate?   *Yes* ❑   *No* ❑

14. Do you have a burning sensation when you urinate?   *Yes* ❑   *No* ❑

    Yes ❑   *No* ❑

15. Is your urine ever dark or cloudy?

    Yes ❑   *No* ❑

16. Is there ever blood in your urine?

17. Do you have chronic pain in your lower back or pelvis?   *Yes* ❑   *No* ❑

18. Do you ever wet yourself during the night?   *Yes* ❑   *No* ❑

19. Do you wear sanitary pads or liners to absorb leakage?   *Yes* ❑   *No* ❑

20. Do you urinate more than eight times a day?   *Yes* ❑   *No* ❑

21. Do you have sudden, unexpected urges to urinate?   *Yes* ❑   *No* ❑

22. Have you had a problem with leakage for more than three months?   *Yes* ❑   *No* ❑

23. Do you experience leakage weekly?   *Yes* ❑   *No* ❑

24. Do you experience leakage daily?   *Yes* ❑   *No* ❑

25. Do you experience leakage hourly?   *Yes* ❑   *No* ❑

26. Do you leak urine during sexual activity?   *Yes* ❑   *No* ❑

27. Do you dread having sex or do you avoid it completely because of urinary leakage?   *Yes* ❑   *No* ❑

28. Have you cut back on any of your normal activities, including work and pleasure, because of leaking urine?   *Yes* ❑   *No* ❑

29. Do you ever feel as though your bladder has not emptied completely and then have leakage afterward?   *Yes* ❑   *No* ❑

PART II:
FINDING HELP

6

OVERCOMING THE EMOTIONAL OBSTACLES TO SEEKING HELP

If millions of women have problems with urinary leakage and only one out of five ever seeks medical help, what is preventing the rest of us from speaking up? There are many reasons. Some are personal, some cultural and some are just plain hard to explain. A problem with bladder control is a complicated situation that can be very painful psychologically and hard to deal with, even if you really want help.

Incontinence is difficult to live with because it makes those who suffer from it feel completely alone and isolated. It's not a problem that is easily shared. Some women may keep asking why this is happening to them or question what they have done to deserve it. It doesn't help to blame yourself for your condition, or question your healthcare decisions in the past and how they may have contributed to your present situation.

You should understand that when you can't control your bladder, it's natural for you to feel many upsetting and negative emotions. At times, you may even feel desperate, not knowing what to do or where to turn for answers.

That's why it is so important for you to examine your emotional response to your condition and realize that your feelings, even when completely justified, can actually be preventing you from going out and getting help. Let's look at some of the emotional issues you may be experiencing and talk about how to handle them successfully.

THE EMOTIONAL ISSUES OF INCONTINENCE

"I'm So Embarrassed"

With incontinence, the word that comes up most often is "embarrassment." The discovery that you can no longer control your bladder and prevent urine from leaking out is a source of profound embarrassment. You want to hide from everyone closest to you and, in fact, from the entire world.

As a very young child, you went through toilet training. If you were like most children, you learned from your mother to recognize the urge to use the toilet and how to make sure you got there in time. When you succeeded, she praised you and told you how "good" and how "grown up" you were. As a young child, you were pleased with your progress, proud of the fact that you were no longer a baby needing diapers, and happy that you had your mother's approval.

Before long, recognizing the need to urinate and getting to a bathroom in time became a matter of habit, something you rarely had to think about. As you grew, your brain developed and your muscles strengthened, and you learned to respond to the need to "hold it in" when no bathroom was available.

Within a few years of toilet training, accidents no longer occurred. In your mind, leakage of urine became associated with babies, the declining elderly; and people with serious medical disorders. In our society, the loss of bladder control has very strong negative associations.

Given this mindset, it is easy to understand why we feel so deeply embarrassed if we suddenly begin to leak urine. Sadly, it is this precise feeling of embarrassment that is often the barrier that prevents us from seeking help. We are simply too embarrassed to tell anyone—including our partners, family, close friends, and most of all, our doctors.

If you are suffering silently, it is important to remember that millions of other women share your condition and that it is almost always a result of factors that you can not control without outside help. Chances are that if you get help, your condition will improve or be cured. There is nothing to be embarrassed about.

"I'm Afraid of What This Means"

Bladder problems also make us fearful. We wonder, "Have I begun my decline into old age?" "Is my life going to be over before much longer?" While you may feel young and vigorous in every other way, the fact that you are now leaking urine can cast a shadow over your life.

Why the fear? Unfortunately, most of us falsely believe that loss of bladder control is an inevitable part of growing older. If you have this conviction, especially if you are postmenopausal, you may fail to ask your physician about the causes or treatments for incontinence. Don't fall into this trap. The days are gone when women were told, "There is nothing we can do for you. You will just have to learn to live with it."

Perhaps you have the false idea that the only effective treatment is surgery. The truth is that there are many effective non-invasive and non-surgical treatments for incontinence (see Part Three.) Surgery is usually reserved for the minority of women who have not improved to their own satisfaction using other treatments.

The truth, of course, is the exact opposite of what your fears may tell you. There is a great deal that can be done about your condition and you don't have to live with it. Don't let fear prevent you from learning the facts and getting the help you need.

"I Feel Anxious All The Time"

Incontinence brings about anxiety. When will you lose control next? Will it be while you are giving an important presentation at work in front of your entire staff? Or during lunch in that nice Chinese restaurant with your mother-in-law? While playing bridge at your friends' house Saturday night? Or making love with your partner?

The truth is that with bladder control problems, you simply don't know when the next accident may occur. You may have a minor problem that you cope with by using sanitary pads, or a major problem that makes it difficult for you to leave the house. Whether the problem is small or large, it can always be a cause of anxiety, something you think about all the time. Especially when other people are around.

This constant anxiety is frequently apparent and baffling to the people close to you. Family and friends may approach you, trying to find out what is wrong. And that becomes a further cause of anxiety. What do you tell them? What stories can you come up with that will seem plausible? How can you hide what is really happening?

The need to cope with sudden, unexpected loss of urine and the need to cover it up at all costs can produce powerful negative changes in your life, increasingly isolating you from the activities and people you love. The sad part is that it's all so unnecessary. Current treatments are so effective that it should quickly become unnecessary for you to worry at all about your condition. Once you go for help, you will have the situation well in hand.

"I'm Really Angry! Why Did This Happen to Me?"

It's easy to understand feelings of embarrassment, but you may also find yourself experiencing intense anger. You may ask yourself over and over, "Why is this happening to me? What did I do to deserve this? I always take such good care of myself—eat right, exercise, enjoy my job, have a positive, loving attitude toward myself and everyone else. Why should I have this terrible problem? It's not right!"

Rest assured that thinking like this is very common, especially in recent years with the popularity of the self-help movement in healthcare. It's understandable that many of us believe that we are solely responsible for our physical health and if anything goes wrong, it's our fault. Even though there is much truth to the belief that you have a strong influence on the state of your health, the real picture is not so cut and dried.

Many medical conditions result from situations that you cannot totally control, including those involving genetic factors or tendencies you inherit from your parents that can result in health problems; infectious agents that can invade your body without your knowledge or participation; and the natural consequences of aging, which none of us can completely avoid.

Feeling angry with yourself because you have a medical problem is self-defeating. The only time your anger may be justified is once you finally get help and realize how much time and effort you wasted feeling angry over a problem that has such effective treatments.

"I Feel So Ashamed"

If you feel you are to blame for your condition, you may also experience shame, which is a sense of embarrassment compounded by guilt. You are convinced that you have done something wrong and are being punished. In other words, you feel certain that you are responsible for your health condition and you are desperate to hide your guilt.

If you suffer from low self-esteem to begin with; and are having a problem with the urine leakage, your loss of bladder control can seem like just one more obstacle to deal with in your life. What's even worse, this time it's a really difficult obstacle.

You may begin to review your life, looking for what you did wrong. "I should never have smoked as a teenager," you think. Or, "I overdid the exercising and now my body is permanently damaged." Or, "I should never have had natural childbirth." Or, "I had too much sex and it did something to my insides."

If you experience shame over your incontinence, you are very likely to hide the problem from everyone in your life and worst of all, avoid asking your doctor for help. You may even wait for years or perhaps never ask at all.

So it's important to remember that incontinence:

- Happens to millions of women
- Has physical causes
- Is highly treatable

Shame is also a strong deterrent to your seeking help. You should never feel shame over having this condition. When you know the facts, shame simply can't be justified.

"I'm Always Depressed"

Today, depression is one of our most widely discussed and publicized medical problems and there are a number of effective medications and therapies to treat it. If you feel depressed about your loss of bladder control, taking a pill is not going to cure your condition. Instead, you have to get medical help in order to find out the cause of your incontinence and what type of treatment can cure or alleviate your loss of bladder control—the cause of your depression.

If you believe that your problem with urinary leakage means that you are well on the way to a nursing home, and if you believe that nothing can be done to reverse your condition, of course you will feel depressed!

This kind of depression is based on false ideas and lack of correct information. Following successful treatment, you will probably regret all the time you spent feeling depressed over a condition that has such successful treatments.

"My Sex Life Is a Disaster"

Incontinence can have a devastating effect on your sex life. Like many women, you may not feel comfortable discussing your sexual activities with your doctor and when leakage of urine begins to cause problems, you may remain silent and simply try to "live with it."

When you can't control your bladder, you may begin to feel unfeminine, unattractive, and undesirable, convinced that you are no longer the same woman your partner fell in love with. Your condition can also depress your sex drive, putting a damper on any desire you may experience for sexual activity and physical affection, and placing your relationship in serious difficulty.

Sexuality itself can complicate the situation when you *think* you have a problem with bladder control and you don't. For example, you may notice that when you reach orgasm, you have a strong urge to urinate and at times, you may actually release some urine. But sometimes when that happens, it can be completely normal, because vaginal penetration can put pressure on your bladder and the surrounding muscles. At other times, a leakage of urine can occur simply because you have not fully emptied your bladder prior to sex.

There is also the possibility that the fluid may not be urine at all, but a clear, odorless secretion released from glands within your vagina (see Chapter Three). Again, this is perfectly normal.

Certain sexual positions can also cause you to lose bladder control, especially if you have some degree of pelvic muscle weakness to begin with. For instance, the missionary position, with the man on top, can result in too much pressure on your lower abdomen, making it difficult to prevent urine from seeping out if you have a full or partially full bladder.

Despite all these possibilities, if you experience what you think is a loss of urine during sex, it's very important to inform your physician, since it may be an indication of a medical problem. If it is incontinence, there is definitely help for you and treatment will definitely improve your sex life.

If your treatment is not entirely successful or still in progress, you and your partner can put waterproof sheets on the bed or use protective devices to prevent leakage (see Chapter Fifteen.)

You can also engage in a variety of lovemaking techniques that do not involve intercourse, such as touching, caressing, kissing, oral sex, or using vibrators. With experimentation, you can discover alternatives that will not result in any unwanted leakage of urine.

THE MYTHS AND THE FACTS ABOUT INCONTINENCE

Many times, these myths come from well-meaning friends and relatives. Let's compare some of these myths to the facts:

MYTH	FACT
1. Incontinence is an inevitable part of the aging process.	1. There are many changes to the urinary tract as we age, but none of these changes invariably lead to urinary incontinence.
2. There is no effective treatment for incontinence.	2. There are many effective treatments.
3. The only treatment is surgery.	3. Surgery is usually used only when no other treatment works to your satisfaction.
4. Most healthcare providers don't know anything about it and would be embarrassed if asked about it.	4. Many providers regularly treat incontinence.
5. The only thing you can do is wear pads or take a pill and hope no one finds out.	5. There are many approaches to treating incontinence, and the condition can be greatly improved or even cured, making pills and pads unnecessary.

Taking Control

It is very important for you to realize that help is available. Many cases of incontinence can be cured and many others helped to the point that you can go back to leading an active and fulfilling life, free from all the negative emotions that may have been bothering you for so long.

The key is taking control of your problem: Learn everything you can about it and take immediate, positive action to make all the improvements you can. Millions of women have already done this, and you can, too. So go ahead and take the first step to finding the help that you need and deserve.

Taking Action

You can use the following steps as you make the transition from suffering in silence to speaking up and finding help:

- Take control and admit to yourself that you have a problem.
- Make a firm resolution to get better and to doeverything you need to do to get better.
- Learn all you can about incontinence.
- Don't wait: Discuss your condition with your doctor right now.
- Find the best doctor to treat your problem, either your regular physician or a recommended specialist (see Chapter Seven).
- Educate yourself about all the treatment options (see Part Three), discuss them with your doctor, and decide together which program of treatment is best for you.
- Faithfully follow the program that you and your physician have chosen.
- Do everything you can do to help yourself, including the exercises and lifestyle changes recommended in Part Three.

If you follow these steps, you will definitely take control of your condition and in time, you will invariably see positive results. It's not always easy, but it's always worth the effort.

7

FINDING THE RIGHT DOCTOR

Even though today, physicians know more than ever about the diagnosis and treatment of urinary incontinence, it is still true that not every physician has the knowledge or expertise to diagnose and treat urinary incontinence properly. It is very important for you to find the right doctor to help you get better.

You may have a primary care physician or internist who knows you well and has treated you for many years. Is he or she the right doctor to treat your incontinence? Or is it necessary for you to consult a specialist in order to get a correct diagnosis and effective treatment?

There is no single right answer to these questions. In some cases, your GP (general practitioner) can do an excellent job of treating your condition, but in other cases, you will probably be better off with a specialist.

Treatment with Your Primary Care Doctor

An initial evaluation and treatment of incontinence can usually be done by any number of healthcare professionals, including general internists, family care doctors, physician's assistants, nurse practitioners and nurse specialists. If you have a primary care physician or other healthcare professional you like and trust, your first step should be to discuss your problem with her or him.

If this person feels comfortable treating your condition, you may want to proceed. After all, it is definitely not necessary to go to a specialist for every medical condition. In many cases, you will not need to go to anyone else. However, if your primary care doctor thinks that because of the severity or complexity of your condition, you should see a specialist right away, or if your initial treatment has not been successful and a specialist seems advisable, your doctor can recommend one.

Consulting a Specialist

Some of the medical specialists who treat urinary incontinence in women include:

- Urologists, doctors who specialize in medical conditions of the urogenital systems of both men and women.
- Gynecologists, doctors who specialize in the medical conditions of women, especially those that relate to reproduction.
- Urogynecologists, physicians who specialize in medical conditions of the urogenital systems in women.
- Nurse specialists, physical therapists, and geriatricians (those who specialize in treating the elderly) may also provide effective treatment for incontinence.

The Ideal Doctor

If you are fortunate, your incontinence will be simple to diagnose and treat. However, in many cases, things don't proceed that quickly or easily. Because of the nature of this problem, it takes time to fully diagnose and come up with an individualized treatment plan.

That's why it is so important to find a doctor who is willing to persist in finding the correct cause or causes for your incontinence and who will also be flexible in trying different approaches until the best solution is found. It may take some time, research, and perseverance to find the doctor who is right for you, but your search will definitely be worth the effort.

Organizations to Contact

There are some excellent organizations providing information and support for those suffering from bladder control problems, and some of them can provide significant help with your search for the right doctor. They include:

American Urological Association and American Foundation for Urologic Disease
877-379-5433 (or 877-DRYLIFE)
Internet: www.drylife.org.
Special database of member urologists who treat incontinence

National Association for Continence (NAFC)
864-579 7900
P.O. Box 8310, Spartanburg, SC 29305-8310
Internet: www.nafc.org
NOTE: this organization was formerly known as H.I.P. (Help for Incontinent People)
Database of health care providers by geographical area, and information on incontinence.

These organizations and others providing information and support for those with bladder control problems are more fully described in Appendix A.

Other Referral Sources

Apart from your primary care physician and the organizations in Appendix A, there are other avenues you can use for obtaining referrals to doctors who treat urinary incontinence.

- A friend or relative who has been treated for incontinence is one of the best sources for finding a good doctor. However, since many people are sensitive about this condition, you may not know any women who will discuss their condition with you. If you do know someone, she can be an excellent source for a referral.

- Your HMO or health insurance company may be able to provide you with a list of member specialists in your area.

- Support groups are often a wonderful source for finding the right doctor in your neighborhood, as well as a source of comfort and support for you while undergoing treatment. You can find more information on incontinence support groups in Chapter Seventeen and in Appendix A at the end of this book.

- The internet can be another good place to find specialists in treating urinary incontinence who are located in your area. Some physician websites also provide detailed information about incontinence and its treatment. However, do not believe everything you see on the Internet. Remember that, unlike a medical journal, no proof of a claim or statement is required. Always proceed with extreme caution.

- The yellow pages of your local telephone book often list specialists in your area. Some physicians and clinics may also have display ads. These ads and those in local newspapers may help you find the right doctor.

- Local hospitals, clinics, and medical colleges may be able to refer you to physicians who specialize in incontinence in your area.

- Books written by medical experts on incontinence may be another source. If the physician author is in your area, you might want to consult him or her. If not, you could call his/her medical office and ask for a referral.

- Companies that make products and medications to treat incontinence sometimes have a list of regional specialists. Contact them through the addresses, phone numbers, and websites printed on their products.

- Medical societies that deal primarily with incontinence and other bladder and urethral problems can be useful resources, but they are usually available only to your doctor. Membership in these societies generally requires that an individual physician possess some special expertise, knowledge or interest in the subject. For specialists in urinary incontinence and related disorders, these include; The Society for Urodynamics and Female Urology (SUFU), The American Urogynecologic Society (AUGS), The International Urogynecological Association (IUGA), and The International Continence Society (ICS).

You can ask your primary care doctor if he or she has access to these organizations and can obtain a referral for you.

If you use your imagination and do a bit of research, you will find many ways to seek out referrals for the best doctor in your area to treat your condition.

You may narrow your list of potential doctors down to just one who has been recommended by several sources, or perhaps there may be two or three whom you want to consider.

Before you make your first appointment or select your doctor, contact each candidate's office to see if you can have a consultation with the doctor. Some insurance plans pay for this type of visit. If yours does not, ask the cost before scheduling an appointment. In some cases, a consultation will be possible, but in other cases, you may have to talk with someone in the office. The goal here is to ask key questions to determine whether this physician is right for you. To help you do this, we have included a list of questions below.

You may not feel completely comfortable asking a doctor or a member of the office staff some of the questions below, but the information you get will be well worth the effort in helping you determine if this doctor is the right one for you. If the doctor or office staff is not willing to take the time to answer your questions, that may also be a factor in your decision.

QUESTIONS TO ASK PROSPECTIVE DOCTORS

When you talk to a prospective doctor or a member of the office staff, your questions should focus on getting information about the doctor's experience, training, background, and general approach to treating incontinence in women.

Experience in Treating Incontinence in Women

- Do you provide treatment for women with incontinence? Obviously, you are looking for a "yes."

- How long have you been treating incontinence? Someone who has more experience may be preferable, but experience alone does not determine the best doctor for your condition. Sometimes a younger doctor may be more versed in newer methods, treatments, and medications. Experience is only one factor—but it can be an important one when you are weighing the differences between two or more candidates.

- Have you treated many women with this problem? Again, someone who has a great deal of experience with this condition may be preferable to one who has less.

• Do you have special equipment to test bladder function (urodynamics) and find the cause of urinary incontinence? If the answer is "yes," it indicates that this physician is familiar with treating incontinence, probably sees many people with the condition, and is sufficiently dedicated to finding its cause to invest in specialized equipment.

Background and training:

• Do you have any special training in treating incontinence in women? A physician who seeks out special training is usually more experienced and knowledgeable about this condition and probably considers its treatment an important part of practicing medicine.

• Do you belong to any of the special medical societies, such as SUFU, AUGS, IUGA, or ICS? Membership in one of these societies indicates a special interest in bladder conditions, including incontinence.

• Have you written any articles or books about incontinence? If the answer is "yes," that can indicate a special interest and expertise in treating this condition.

Approach to Treatment

• Do you work with any other specialists? Which ones? Why? If the answer is "yes," it may indicate that the doctor makes referrals to other specialists in order to gather as much information as possible for proper diagnosis and treatment.

• Do you offer different options including behavioral therapies and inserts, in addition to surgical procedures? If the answer is "yes," it indicates that the doctor will work with you in order to find the best course of treatment for your individual condition, including the less invasive and less costly approaches.

Remember that the information you gather about a potential doctor needs to be evaluated. Someone who has a great deal of experience and expertise may not necessarily be the best physician for you. The choice you make about the doctor you want to treat you is an individual one. By gathering as much information as you can and evaluating it in terms of your unique needs, you will be better equipped to make your choice.

Also remember that if you are not happy with your doctor, or feel you need greater expertise to successfully treat your condition, you can always go to someone else later on. Never allow your uncertainty to be an excuse for not getting any treatment at all.

QUESTIONS TO ASK BEFORE YOUR FIRST VISIT TO THE DOCTOR'S OFFICE

You can usually save quite a lot of time by asking the doctor's office to send you information and forms prior to your first visit. You can also learn something about how the doctor's office functions and what kinds of services are provided. The following questions will help you to focus on what specific information you should request.

- *Can you send me any printed material about incontinence?* If such information is readily available, it will tell you that the doctor regularly treats people with your condition and wants them to be educated about it.

- *What information should I bring for my first visit?* By knowing about this in advance, you can arrive well prepared with the data your physician needs in order to help you. You can also avoid having to take forms home to get missing information and then having to remember to return them to the office once the information has been located.

- *Do you have a questionnaire that I can fill out in advance?* Some medical offices have a special questionnaire covering information on the patient's history of urinary problems and factors that may be related to it (see sample in Chapter Eight). By bringing a completed questionnaire with you to your first visit, you will save time and perhaps be able to begin your visit sooner. You will also be certain that all the information the physician needs is readily available.

• *Are you a member of my HMO or do you accept my medical insurance?* You will want to know this in advance, so you will not be surprised by any bills that your health insurance company will not cover.

By asking these questions, getting needed forms and information, and preparing for your first medical visit, you will arrive for your appointment feeling better informed and more confident—ready to begin your journey to better health.

8

PREPARING FOR YOUR FIRST MEDICAL VISIT

Your first medical visit is very important. If you arrive well prepared, you can help both yourself and your doctor to find the cause of your condition and the most effective treatment to improve and possibly cure it.

BE PATIENT IF YOU HAVE A COMPLICATED, SEVERE, OR LONG-STANDING CONDITION

As you are now aware, not every doctor has extensive training and experience with treating female incontinence. Even those who do can find it difficult at times to arrive at the correct diagnosis.

You have seen how many different factors and conditions can cause urinary leakage and you also understand that it is possible for you to have more than one type of incontinence and more than one cause for your condition.

That is why it may be important to find a physician who has expertise in treating your condition, especially if it is long-standing and severe, and to work patiently with him or her until a successful solution is found.

You will be very disappointed and discouraged if you anticipate an immediate cure, so remember not to expect too much too soon. Many times, treating incontinence requires trying out different treatments and approaches until the right one is found. A doctor is not a magician and can't always pinpoint the precise cause of your condition instantly.

When you find a doctor you like, follow his or her instructions, remain patient, and remember that just as your incontinence problem did not come about overnight, it may not go away in a short time either. If you stick to your treatment program, you should ultimately be very satisfied with the results.

MEDICAL QUESTIONNAIRE

When you go for your first medical visit, take the completed questionnaire you requested when you made your appointment. Even if your doctor doesn't have a questionnaire, it's still a good idea to bring the following information about yourself and your condition that might be useful in helping the doctor make an accurate diagnosis.

On page XXX in this chapter, you will find a sample questionnaire that is based on one used by physicians who specialize in treating incontinence. We suggest you photocopy it, fill it in, and take it along on your first visit. The questionnaire contains detailed questions that should be of help to any physician. If you decide not to use the questionnaire, bring detailed lists of the following information to make it easier for you in filling out the forms in the doctor's office, or even just to use in your initial discussion. In order to make an accurate diagnosis, physicians take your whole personal history into account, so be ready with the answers.

INFORMATION TO BRING ALONG

Lists of:

- All prescription medications you take, including hormones (estrogens)
- All over-the-counter drugs you use
- All vitamins or other supplements you take
- Foods you eat regularly
- Surgical operations you have had
- Injuries, illnesses, and hospitalizations
- Which recreational drugs you use or have used
- How many times you have given birth, noting if the births were vaginal, caesarian, breech, or otherwise difficult
- Prior treatments or surgeries for incontinence and how well they worked, along with any previous doctor's office records or hospital records documenting prior treatments or surgeries for incontinence and copies of reports on any urinary tract or pelvic x-rays
- Allergies
- Major illnesses in family members

Information on:

- If you have a problem with constipation
- Whether or not you smoke or have smoked in the past.
- How much and what type of alcoholic beverages you consume weekly

A SAMPLE QUESTIONNAIRE

The following is a sample of an incontinence questionnaire that is used by many physicians who regularly treat this condition. Make a photocopy, fill it out, and take it with you on your first visit. It will help you in your initial discussion with the doctor.

Name _____   Date _____

VOIDING HISTORY

1. How many times do you get up at night because you have to urinate?

2. Please fill in the frequency or number of times you need to urinate during the day:

   Between morning and lunchtime: _____
   Between lunchtime and dinnertime: _____
   Between dinnertime and bedtime: _____

3. Do you experience urinary urgency (a sudden need to get to the bathroom)?   *Yes* ❏   *No* ❏

4. When you feel the urge to urinate, are you unable to postpone or suppress it?   *Yes* ❏   *No* ❏

5. What will happen if you are unable to get to the bathroom?   *Pain* ❏ *Pressure* ❏   *Leakage* ❏ *Other:* _____

6. Do you leak urine on the way to the bathroom at night?   *Yes* ❏   *No* ❏

7. Do you feel an *obstruction* to the flow of urine?   *Yes* ❑   *No* ❑

8. Do you have to push or strain in order to start urinating?   *Yes* ❑   *No* ❑

9. Does it take a long time for you to start urinating?   *Yes* ❑   *No* ❑

10. Do you feel that you do not empty your bladder well after urinating?   *Yes* ❑   *No* ❑

11. Do you feel that you have a decreased force of urinary stream when urinating?   *Yes* ❑   *No* ❑

12. Do you leak urine involuntarily (incontinence) during the day?   *Yes* ❑   *No* ❑

13. If yes: How many pads or liners per day do you use?   *Yes* ❑   *No* ❑

14. How wet are they when you change?
Soaked   ❑
Wet   ❑
Damp   ❑
Mostly Dry   ❑

15. Under which of the following circumstances do you leak urine?

   ❑ *Coughing, sneezing, laughing, lifting, standing exercise.*
   ❑ *Because you can't get to the bathroom fast enough.*
   ❑ *Leak constantly all the time.*
   ❑ *Other (please explain):* _____

   _____

   _____

   _____

16. Do you wet the bed while lying down in bed at night?   *Yes* ❑   *No* ❑

17. Have you ever received treatment of any kind for your leakage?   *Yes* ❑   *No* ❑

18. If yes, please explain type of treatment (pills, surgery, exercises, etc.)

_____

_____

19. Approximately how many glasses (8–10 oz.) of fluid (water, soda, beer, wine, coffee, etc.) do you drink in the course of an average day?   ____

20. Do you have pain when you urinate?   *Yes* ❑   *No* ❑
    If yes, please explain:_____

_____

21. Do you have pain relieved by urinating?   *Yes* ❑   *No* ❑

22. Have you ever seen blood in your urine or been told that you have blood in the urine?   *Yes* ❑   *No* ❑

23. Have you ever had a urinary tract infection (bladder, kidney, etc.)?   *Yes* ❑   *No* ❑
    If yes, please explain:

_____

_____

24. Have you ever had a kidney, bladder or ureteral stone?   *Yes* ❑   *No* ❑

If yes, please explain:

_____

_____

_____

25. Have you ever had a cancer of the urinary
    tract (kidney, bladder, etc.)   *Yes* ❏   *No* ❏

    If yes, please explain:

    _____

    _____

    _____

26. How many times have you been pregnant?   _____

27. How many children have you had by   _____
    vaginal delivery?

28. How many children have you had by   _____
    caesarean section ("C" section)?

    How long ago was your last delivery?   _____

29. Were any of the deliveries especially   *Yes* ❏   *No* ❏
    difficult?

    If yes, please explain:

    _____

    _____

    _____

30. Are you still having menstrual periods? *Yes* ❏   *No* ❏

31. If yes, are you menstruating today?   *Yes* ❏   *No* ❏

32. Have you had a hysterectomy (removal   *Yes* ❏   *No* ❏
    of the uterus or womb?)

33. If yes, why was the hysterectomy done
    (i.e. cancer, bleeding, fibroid tumors, etc.)?

    _____

    _____

    _____

34. Was the hysterectomy done through the   _____
    abdomen or the vagina?

35. Were the ovaries removed at the same   *Yes* ❏   *No* ❏
    time?

36. Were any other surgical procedures   *Yes* ❏   *No* ❏
    done at the same time?

    If yes, please describe:

    _____

    _____

    _____

37. Are you presently taking any female   *Yes* ❏   *No* ❏
    hormone replacements?

    If yes, what type (pills, creams, patch)?

    _____

    _____

    _____

    If yes, for how long have you been taking
    estrogen therapy?

    _____

    _____

40. When was your last complete gyneco-
logic (internal) examination and Pap
smear?

_____

41. When was your last mammogram?

_____

42. Have you been diagnosed with   *Yes* ❑   *No* ❑
endometriosis?

The actual questionnaire you receive in your doctor's office may be
different from this one. It may require more information or less information. But if you bring the above information with you, it will definitely be helpful to your physician.

Your Voiding Diary

Below is a sample voiding or bladder diary for one day. You can make
multiple copies of this form and fill one out for two or three days prior
to your first medical appointment, or you can ask your doctor's office
if they have their own form that they want you to use. The voiding
diary will be your personal record of urination over two or three days
and will give your doctor important information about the details of
your medical condition.

You will be asked to record the time of day each time you urinate;
the exact amount of urine you void; the exact amount of fluid you
drink; the types of fluid you drink; whether you have any urgency or
pain before voiding; and whether there is any leakage of urine prior to
voiding.

Always use a measuring cup to record the exact amount or volume
of urine produced throughout the day and night each time you uri-

nate. Be sure to be as accurate as possible in recording the amount of each urination, as well as the time of the day for each urination.

Bring your completed voiding diary to your first visit with the doctor. With the information obtained from this record, you and your doctor may be able to find a pattern to your incontinence which will help to indicate which type or types you have and what further tests you may require.

VOIDING DIARY

Time of Day	Amount Voided (oz. or cc.)	Amount Fluid Intake (drinks)	Type of Fluid Consumed (water, coffee, soda, beer, etc.)	Urgency or pain prior to voiding? (Yes/No)	Leakage of urine at any time prior to voiding? (Yes/No)
7:00 A.M.					
8:00					
9:00					
10:00					
11:00					
12:00 P.M.					
1:00					
2:00					
3:00					
4:00					
5:00					
6:00					
7:00					
8:00					
9:00					
10:00					
11:00					
12:00 A.M.					
1:00					
2:00					
3:00					
4:00					
5:00					
6:00					

YOUR FIRST MEDICAL VISIT

Now that you have gathered a great deal of detailed information about your health and the factors that may be contributing to your incontinence, you are ready for your first visit to the doctor to evaluate your condition.

THE MEDICAL HISTORY FORM

When you go to the doctor's office for your first visit, you will be asked to fill out a detailed medical history form if you have not seen this physician before. This form includes details about your current medical condition, past medical problems and surgeries, and general information, such as your age, occupation, and marital status. This data about your life and your medical history supplement the information provided on the incontinence questionnaire and voiding diary, and can help the doctor pinpoint the cause of your bladder problem.

YOUR FIRST MEETING WITH THE DOCTOR

When you meet with the doctor, you may sit in the office first and discuss your bladder control problem and then have a physical examination, or the doctor may give you the physical examination first and talk with you afterward. The average time for this first office visit is about twenty minutes.

The doctor will review the information provided on the incontinence questionnaire, voiding diary, and medical history form covering your life, habits, medical history and current condition. Then the doctor will ask you some questions. When you answer, try to provide as much information as possible, since there are many different clues to the origins of bladder control problems. Sometimes information you may think is not important can actually be vital when making a diagnosis. Topics that may be discussed with your doctor include:

- How long you have had the problem
- How it has affected your social life
- How it has affected your marriage, your sex life, and your other important relationships
- How you deal with the condition
- Whether other women in your family have had the same problem
- Any ideas you might have about what could be causing your incontinence.
- Any previous doctors you have seen for incontinence and any treatments you have tried in the past

9

HOW INCONTINENCE IS DIAGNOSED

Your doctor will go through a number of steps in the process of making a diagnosis. While some cases can be quickly diagnosed and successfully treated, most require a few diagnostic tests and several different approaches before the condition improves or goes away altogether. For successful therapy, patience is a must.

As you discuss your bladder control problem during the initial consultation, your physician will also be assessing your mental state and determining whether you have such problems as impaired memory, which can affect urinary function.

You will also be observed carefully for any signs of neurological problems which can be linked to incontinence. A droopy eye, a limp, a facial tic, or other signs may be present and you may not even be aware of them.

Diagnostic Tests

After your initial visit, your doctor will study the results of your physical exam, medical history, and voiding diary. At that point, he or she may have an idea about what type of incontinence you have and what is causing it. The next step is to decide which tests you need.

Some of the tests described below may be used routinely by primary care physicians, while others are used only by specialists, such as urologists. So depending on your individual condition and your doctor's specialty, you may or may not be given the tests described here.

The Physical Exam

A thorough physical examination will give further clues about the type and severity of your incontinence. The physician or nurse specialist may perform a *cotton swab test,* in which a lubricated cotton swab (like a Q-Tip) is inserted in your urethra. When you cough, the movement of the swab helps determine the position of your bladder and whether your urethra is slipping out of place when you move, as is the case in some women with stress incontinence. Although there is no pain with this test, it creates the sensation of needing to urinate and may be slightly uncomfortable for that reason.

A *pelvic exam* can, in some cases, reveal weakened pelvic floor muscles, hormonal deficiency (loss of estrogen, especially after menopause), or a prolapsed bladder or uterus.

An examination of the front (anterior) vaginal wall can determine whether you have a prolapse and if you have hypermobility of the urethra or a prolapsed bladder called a cystocele (see Chapter Fourteen.)

Finally, a *digital rectal exam,* in which (the doctor's gloved finger is inserted into your rectum, can help to determine your muscle strength, including your pelvic floor muscles.

Your first physical examination will take approximately five to ten minutes and may involve some minor discomfort when your doctor uses a speculum to examine your vagina or performs the digital rectal exam.

The diagnostic tests described below are presented in order of invasiveness, with the simplest, least invasive tests first and the more invasive tests later on.

Pad Tests

With this test, you are given sanitary pads to wear for a twenty-four hour period, changing them whenever necessary. As each pad is removed, it is stored in a sealed plastic bag. After the test period ends, the used pads are returned to the doctor's office where they are weighed to measure the amount of urine leaked, giving your doctor an idea of how much urine you are losing daily. This test can be very useful and important in making an accurate diagnosis, as well as for comparing the amount of leakage before and after any treatment.

Urine Tests

Urine testing can often reveal infections or even tumors which may be linked to urinary incontinence. You'll have to provide only a urine sample, so there is no discomfort involved. There are several different types of urine tests.

Urinalysis is often used to diagnose a bladder infection or cystitis. This test, also known as a dipstick test, can also reveal whether or not you have blood or sugar in your urine, and whether large amounts of harmful bacteria are present. It can be performed in your doctor's office and the results are known almost immediately.

Culture and sensitivity tests can identify the presence of specific types of harmful bacteria, so your doctor can determine what medication to prescribe. For this test, your urine will be sent to a medical laboratory and the results will be known in one or two days.

Urodynamic Tests

Urodynamic tests refer to a group of diagnostic procedures that determine how your bladder and sphincter muscle are functioning during the filling, storing, and emptying phases of the urinary process. This information can help to pinpoint what type of incontinence you have and will also determine the appropriate treatment. Urodynamic tests are often used for women with mixed symptoms and for those who are more difficult to diagnose. These procedures help reveal whether the bladder and sphincter muscle are working properly:

Uroflowmetry

This is a test to measure and record the amount of urine that leaves your bladder and how quickly it is expelled. In this test, you simply urinate into a special commode. Since this test is not invasive, there is no pain or discomfort involved and it should only take about three or four minutes to complete. No catheterization or other manipulation is required. This test measures how quickly the detrusor muscle pushes urine out of the bladder. It may also suggest whether a blockage is present in the urethra.

Post-Void Residual Urine Measurement

Post-void residual urine measurement is a test to measure the urine that remains in your bladder after you have urinated.

This procedure can be done either by *ultrasound*, a non-invasive, but costly procedure, that takes about two minutes and is pain-free; or *catheterization*, which is more accurate, but is also invasive and may be mildly uncomfortable.

Elderly women suffering from recurring urinary tract infections; women with complicated neurological diseases; and women who do not seem to be emptying their bladders properly can benefit from this type of test.

Cystometry

This is a test to measure how effectively your bladder stores and releases urine, as well as the sensations you experience as your bladder fills up and empties. In this test, a small pressure-measuring catheter is inserted into your bladder and sometimes, with more complex cystometry equipment, a pressure-measuring catheter is also inserted into the rectum. These probes monitor changes in pressure while your bladder is filling up and emptying.

You may feel some slight discomfort or pain during this test. Most commonly, the insertion of a catheter may merely give you an "unusual" sensation, which does not involve any discomfort. As your bladder fills, you will also feel a desire to urinate. It is important to tell the doctor or nurse doing the test if you feel pain, because you shouldn't feel any. Cystometry takes between five and ten minutes to complete.

Leak Point Pressure or Urethral Pressure Profile

This is a test that measures how well your urethral sphincter muscle is functioning. This test is part of cystometry and is almost never performed separately. After the small cystometry catheter is inserted into the bladder and the bladder is filled to a certain point, the patient coughs, generating pressure in the bladder. In women with stress incontinence, this cough may be sufficient to force urine out of the urethra. The leak point pressure test measures the pressure at which urine leaks out of the urethra. The lower the leak point pressure, the worse the stress incontinence.

Cystography or Voiding Cystourethrogram (VCUG)

This is an X ray of your bladder and urethra in which your bladder is filled via a catheter with a special fluid that can be seen on an X ray. X rays are taken during the filling of your bladder, during straining and coughing, and during urination.

You may feel some discomfort when the catheter is inserted. This test takes about twenty minutes to complete.

Videourodynamics

This is a highly specialized test which combines cystometry, uroflowmetry, and cystography. All the tests are combined and done at the same time. In this test, very special small probes are placed into your bladder and rectum, permitting the most sophisticated diagnostic evaluation of your bladder and urethra currently available. Videourodynamics is the best and most definitive test for determining the type and causes of even the most complicated kinds of incontinence. This test involves the insertion of the same general type of catheters as used in cystometry. The major advantage of videourodynamics is that it combines several tests which are done at the same time with no additional discomfort or cost. The disadvantages are that the equipment required to do it is very expensive, not widely available, and it must be interpreted by a specialist or an expert in the field. This test takes from ten to twenty minutes to complete.

Intravenous Urogram (IVU)

This involves a dye test and X ray which evaluates the structure and function of your kidneys and ureters. This test involves injecting a dye into a vein your arm, takes about thirty minutes to complete, and is not painful.

Ultrasound

This is a simple, non-invasive test which uses sound waves to evaluate the structure of your kidneys or bladder. Ultrasound takes about thirty minutes to complete and involves no pain or discomfort.

Cystoscopy

Cystoscopy involves the use of a small, thin telescope that has a light on the end and allows your doctor to see into your urethra and the inside of your bladder.

A good view of your bladder can sometimes reveal the presence of bladder tumors or stones, which can create blockage to the flow of urine. Using cystoscopy, the doctor is also able to remove a small sample of bladder tissue (biopsy) if needed.

Cystoscopy takes from five to ten minutes to complete. You may feel like you need to urinate during cystoscopy, but it should not be painful. The use of newer, smaller instruments has made it less likely that you will feel any discomfort or pain during this procedure.

Making a Diagnosis

Following completion of all the recommended tests and an evaluation of their results, your physician should be able to diagnose your condition and tell you what type or types of incontinence you have, and give you a good idea of what specific treatment may help to alleviate or possibly cure your condition.

If your diagnosis and subsequent treatment do not result in improvement in your urinary incontinence within a reasonable period of time (also see Chapter Seventeen), you may want to ask if additional testing might be helpful, since it is possible that the primary cause or additional causes of your bladder control problem may not have been identified.

Underlying Conditions Causing Incontinence

One of the main reasons you should see a doctor for immediate diagnosis is to identify any underlying conditions that may be causing your urinary incontinence, so they can be treated and not allowed to progress and get worse.

Some of the underlying diseases that can contribute to incontinence are:

- diabetes
- spinal tumors
- bladder cancer
- neurological diseases, including Parkinson's disease,multiple sclerosis, Alzheimer's disease and stroke.

In most people without any other symptoms or problems, finding such underlying conditions as a the cause of urinary incontinence is rare, so there is no need to be unduly worried when you go to see your physician for the first appointment. The chances are quite good that your condition will have a diagnosis and treatment that will lead to rapid improvement and will not uncover any major health problems, but as with all diseases, early diagnosis is the key to a successful treatment and cure.

PART THREE:
TREATING INCONTINENCE

IO:

GENERAL TREATMENTS FOR INCONTINENCE

You will be amazed how many treatments are available for urinary incontinence, including:

- Lifestyle changes
- Dietary changes
- Changes in medication
- Psychotherapy

- Kegel exercises
- Biofeedback
- Timed voiding
- Bladder retraining
- Electrical stimulation
- Vaginal weights or cones
- Urethral insert devices
- Pessaries
- Self-catheterization
- Collagen injections
- Hormone replacement therapy
- Other medications
- Various forms of surgery

Most women are treated with a combination of therapies and progress gradually toward regaining bladder control. Sometimes the initial treatment doesn't work and others are then prescribed. An experienced doctor is not in a hurry and will work with you until the cause of your bladder control problem is identified and your condition improved to your satisfaction by the most effective therapies.

THE NON-TREATMENT OPTION

Not everybody who has urinary incontinence wants or needs treatment. For example, there are some women who don't want treatment for their bladder control problems and only consult a doctor to get an evaluation and reassurance that they have no serious underlying medical problem.

Other women may have minimal amounts of urinary leakage and are not terribly bothered by it. They may not want any therapy, either. Even so, it is very important to realize that the amount of incontinence or the number of incontinence episodes you experience are not necessarily the major factors in determining whether you decide to get treatment.

The actual volume of urine that you leak is really not that important when deciding whether or not to have treatment. If you don't have any of the serious underlying medical problems previously mentioned, the main factor that will decide whether or not you want to pursue treatment should be the degree of bother to you from your condition, not the amount of leakage.

Making this decision is very subjective and has to be determined on an individual basis. For example, a few drops of urinary incontinence may be tolerable to one woman, but those same few drops may be incapacitating to another woman.

On the other hand, some women can tolerate soaking six, eight, ten, or even twelve pads a day with urine and aren't terribly bothered by it at all. Only you can decide how much your condition affects you and whether or not you want to seek treatment to improve it. However, in some people with underlying problems such as urinary tract cancer, stones, or complications related to the incontinence, such as skin breakdown or infections, treatment is essential.

Guidelines for Treatment Selection

With so many different possibilities, how do you and your doctor decide whether or not you want to have treatment and if so, which one(s)? There are several factors you will want to consider.

• *Start with the most conservative and least invasive treatment first.* In that way, there are lower costs, fewer side effects, and less potential complications. However, for some women, conservative, non-invasive therapy may not be desirable or advisable as a first-line therapy.

• *Choose the treatment appropriate for the type of incontinence.* Certain treatments work best for stress incontinence, others for urge incontinence, and other treatments can be effective for several types of bladder problems (see Chapters Eleven through Fourteen.) Select the type of treatment that is appropriate for your diagnosis. For example, if you have a very low level of estrogen, and thinning tissues are suspected as a factor in your incontinence, you might want to consider hormone replacement. But for other women with a different diagnosis, this therapy might not be effective.

- *Consider the degree of bother to you from your incontinence.* If you only have a mild degree of bother, you may decide to try less invasive methods first. But if your condition is really troubling and your life is miserable as a result, you may want to consider surgery right away if it is appropriate for your condition (it is often helpful for stress incontinence, but rarely for urge incontinence).

- *Choose surgery only when truly indicated, or when nothing else works to your satisfaction.* Surgery is the most expensive, the most invasive, and the most complex of all the treatments for urinary incontinence and should only be selected when you and your doctor have determined that it is the best option.

YOUR ATTITUDE TOWARD TREATMENT

Remember that whatever treatment or treatments you and your physician select, success will largely depend on how well you follow instructions and how faithfully you stick to your program. It is also important to be realistic in your expectations and not to anticipate an instant cure. You should also remind yourself that you are unique and the treatment that works well for another woman may not work at all for you.

II

BEHAVIORAL TECHNIQUES

Behavioral techniques are non-invasive or minimally invasive approaches designed to help you adjust your lifestyle and change the way you behave in relation to urination. They help you adjust your liquid intake, learn to urinate more often, recognize when your bladder is about to contract or when you are about to leak, and strengthen the muscles involved in preventing urination. These approaches require that you follow a specific program in order to see results.

For some women, the effects of behavioral therapies can be augmented with additional devices, equipment or therapies (see Chapters

Eleven and Fifteen.) Although they vary in effectiveness, some of these devices can be expensive or rarely, even relatively invasive.

HOW BEHAVIORAL TECHNIQUES CAN HELP YOU

In most cases, it is a good idea to begin with one or more behavioral techniques to see if they improve or even cure your incontinence. That is why behavioral techniques are usually the first line of treatment for incontinence, especially in mild to moderate cases. Then, if these techniques are not successful, you can go on to other forms of therapy. In some cases, these behavioral techniques are used in conjunction with medication, since these two forms of treatment are easily combined.

Scientific studies on behavioral techniques are quite positive, showing very good results for women who follow them properly. Some studies of these techniques indicate that the incidence of incontinence and the amount of urine lost during incontinent episodes have shown reductions of more than 50 percent when the techniques are properly followed.

Many healthcare professionals are not well-informed about all the different types of behavioral techniques, although this situation has been showing signs of improvement recently. Overall, these therapies require an investment of time and effort. Positive results are generally seen only after several weeks to months. However, with some patience, these behavioral techniques can be effective, lifelong solutions which are relatively non-invasive, low-cost treatments with almost no adverse effects.

LIFESTYLE CHANGES

Sometimes, easy changes in your lifestyle can be helpful in combatting incontinence. Here are some examples of helpful lifestyle changes you can make—even if you do not have bladder control problems, these changes are good for your overall health and can also help prevent future incontinence.

Stop smoking

Smokers frequently develop a cough, and this chronic coughing weakens the pelvic floor muscles. In addition, smoking can cause damage to parts of the urinary system, including the bladder and urethra. In fact, smoking causes many changes in body tissues and results in a systemic problem which is not limited to the urinary tract. Tissue damage caused by smoking can injure the heart, lungs, bladder, urethra, and many other parts of the body. If you are a smoker, you should take immediate steps to put a permanent to stop this habit which can be so devastating to your health.

Lose weight

Excess poundage puts additional stress on the bladder and pelvic floor muscles, which may lead to urinary leakage.

Exercise regularly

As you know, a sedentary lifestyle is not healthy and often results in added weight. When you follow a regular exercise program, it will help keep you trim and will also strengthen your muscles, including the ones that are important for proper urinary function.

Changes in Diet

You have seen how certain foods and drinks may be irritants to your urinary system (see Chapter Three). These substances include caffeinated coffee and tea, alcohol, carbonated beverages (with or without caffeine), milk and milk products, citrus juice and citrus fruits, tomatoes and tomato products, chocolate, sugar, honey, corn syrup, artificial sweeteners (aspartame, saccharin), and very spicy foods.

While many women have no problems with any of these items, other women do. In some women, one or more of these foods or beverages may stimulate the bladder and result in urinary incontinence.

In fact, some women may find that by giving up caffeine and alcohol, two of the most frequent culprits, they can significantly improve or even eliminate mild symptoms of incontinence.

However, giving up caffeine and alcohol may not be as simple as it sounds. You may not be aware that these substances are sometimes ingredients in products you use regularly, such as cough and cold preparations and other over-the-counter medications. For that reason, it is important for you to carefully read the labels before using any product you ingest.

You should also be aware that alcohol can damage a number of tissues in the body that affect the urinary cycle, including the brain, nerves, and bladder tissue itself, causing negative effects on the urinary tract. Excessive alcohol consumption can definitely make your bladder problems much worse.

Another common offender is sugar, not just in its white refined form, but also in other forms such as honey, corn syrup, and brown sugar. Even sugar substitutes can have an adverse effect on the bladder and should be avoided if they are found to be a problem.

Like caffeine and alcohol, sugar is often a hidden ingredient in many prepared foods and over-the-counter medications, so once again, it is important for you to carefully check the label before using them.

How do you know if any of these foods are related to your incontinence? One good way to find out is to keep a "food diary" for a week. Record everything you eat and drink and every medication you take for one week, keeping track of the time you take each item. Then record the times when you urinate and the episodes of urinary incontinence (see Voiding Diary, Chapter Eight). After a week, see if you can find a connection between using one or more items and your urinary leakage.

Of course, it is a good idea to evaluate your food diary under the supervision of your physician. If you find that certain items seem to be causing trouble, you can substitute something else. For example, you can use carob instead of chocolate, or decaffeinated coffee and herbal teas instead of those with caffeine.

Another problem that involves diet and incontinence is constipation. When you habitually strain in the bathroom during bowel movements, you can weaken your pelvic floor, causing or exacerbating your incontinence. A diet that is high in fiber and has sufficient liquids can be helpful. If that is not sufficient, stool softeners or natural laxatives such as psyllium can also be helpful. You should discuss these options with your doctor.

Changes in Medication

We have already seen that many prescription drugs and over-the-counter medications have been linked with urinary incontinence (see Chapter Three). If you take any of these drugs, it is important to find out if they may be the cause, or one of the causes, of your urinary incontinence.

These drugs include certain antihistamines, sedatives, muscle relaxants, diuretics, anticholinergics, calcium channel blockers, antidepressants, and narcotics.

If you read the package insert, you should find urinary incontinence listed as one of the possible side effects. Of course, these substances do not cause incontinence in every woman who uses them, but they may be contributing to the problem in your case.

If your doctor has prescribed one of these medications, you should never stop taking it on your own, even if you suspect it may be causing your loss of bladder control. The connection between the drug and urinary problems is something you need to discuss with your doctor and if a connection is proven, an alternative drug that is less likely to cause a problem can be prescribed.

Once again, it is a good idea for you to keep a diary for a week, this time recording the exact times when you take your medication and then comparing them with the exact times when you have urinary leakage or an excessive need to urinate. Your doctor will help you to evaluate this diary and find out if there might be a connection between your medication and your bladder control problems.

PSYCHOTHERAPY

Occasionally, psychotherapy is recommended for treating urinary incontinence. In cases where your bladder control problem is connected to depression, anxiety, or phobias, for example, this form of therapy can result in a significant improvement. Of course, it is also true that incontinence caused by physical, or non-psychological, problems can create feelings of depression or anxiety, so it is important to determine which comes first.

Even when psychological difficulties are not the direct cause of incontinence, psychotherapy can often be helpful because it can alleviate the emotional distress that you may experience as a result of this disorder.

When you are feeling better and more in control of yourself and your disorder, you are better equipped to deal with your incontinence and work toward a solution. It is a good idea to discuss the possibility of psychotherapy with your physician if you think it might be useful for you. (See Chapter Sixteen for information on coping with the emotional issues brought about by incontinence).

BEHAVIORAL MODIFICATION

Behavioral modification is an effective program for the management of many types of urinary incontinence, including both stress and urge incontinence. However, it does *not* work for women with overflow incontinence. This program consists of the following:

Education

Simply by rereading Chapter Two, you will have a good understanding of the structure and function of your lower urinary tract. You should realize that your body makes urine all day, every minute of the day. It is the sole function of your bladder to store urine as it accumulates and then, by relaxation of your urinary sphincters and contraction of the detrusor muscle of your bladder, to finish the urinary cycle by emptying to completion.

Fluid Management

A normal, healthy individual makes approximately one to two ounces of urine per hour throughout the day, but this can vary considerably based on the amount of fluids you drink, foods that you eat, activity of the person, the outside temperature, and several other factors. Even so, since urine is composed mostly of water, a healthy person must consume enough fluid (water, juice, etc.) to replace the amount of water lost from the body. Water is lost from the body in many ways other than by urination, including perspiration (sweat), breathing, and defecation (stool).

However, since there is plenty of water and fluid in the foods you eat, replacement fluids do not have to equal the amount of urine produced. Usually, if you drink six to eight-ounce glasses of fluid per day, that is sufficient to provide you with adequate fluid replacement. The information you provide when you properly fill out your voiding diary (see Chapter Eight) will provide an excellent source of information regarding the desirable amount of fluid intake. Remember that everybody is different and has different needs, especially those with other medical illnesses. Thus, all recommendations and guidelines in this book, including fluid intake, should be discussed in detail between you and your doctor, who, after all, knows you the best.

A good rule of thumb is that you should drink enough fluid to produce about thirty to forty ounces of urine over a period of twenty-four hours. If you produce more urine than that in that time, you may be drinking too much fluid. Before you change your daily fluid intake, always check with your physician to make sure that you do not have any medical conditions which require above average fluid intake.

Drinking excessive water or other fluids will simply force your kidneys to make more urine and your bladder to handle more urine. Although it is not necessarily unhealthy to make excessive urine, when you are incontinent, the excess fluid results in more urine accumulating in your bladder quicker, and the result is that you experience more urinary incontinence.

For the greatest improvement with your condition, you should combine proper fluid management with the other parts of a behavioral modification program.

Timed Voiding

Like many women, you may be helped by a timed schedule for going to the toilet. Usually, it involves going every two to four hours, regardless of whether you feel the need to urinate or not.

This type of approach is recommended if you lead a very busy life and often postpone visits to the bathroom, sometimes for hours at a time; if you are physically disabled and require assistance in order to go to the bathroom; and if you have neurological disorders, such as Alzheimer's disease, and do not receive signals that you need to urinate.

If you leak because your bladder contracts without your permission (urge incontinence), the exact frequency of how often timed voiding should be performed can be calculated from your voiding diary: an interval shorter than the usual time between your episodes of urgency. If you have stress incontinence, timed voiding is also effective, since a full bladder will leak more than an almost empty one.

Remember, the underlying principle behind timed voiding is to empty your bladder intermittently on a regular schedule, avoiding the sensation of urinary urgency followed by urgency incontinence. The idea is that if your bladder is constantly emptied there will be little or no urine to leak out.

PRIVATE PRACTICE VIBRATION REMINDER DISK

The Private Practice Vibration Reminder Disk is a useful device that is worn on your body and is preprogrammed to vibrate several times throughout the day. The disk assists you in following the procedures for timed voiding and behavioral modification. In essence, it acts as a gentle reminder to void at various times through the day. It may also assist in your performance of pelvic floor exercises (see sections below). Note that you can achieve the same results at a lower cost by using a wrist watch with an alarm.

BLADDER RETRAINING

Bladder retraining is similar to timed voiding, except that your intervals between visiting the toilet are gradually increased. This approach helps you to recognize the physical signs that you need to urinate. It is used mainly for urge incontinence but it can be helpful with other types of urinary incontinence, as well.

In bladder training protocols, the voiding interval is gradually increased over the course of several weeks to months. A reasonable plan would be perhaps to increase the voiding interval by fifteen minutes at a time every two to three weeks. Use of a voiding diary over this period of time helps to monitor progress. Concomitant and strategic use of pelvic floor exercises in inhibiting bladder overactivity can contribute to a very successful program of bladder retraining (see later discussion on pelvic floor exercises). The goal of bladder retraining is to achieve a reasonable voiding interval while maintaining complete dryness.

Other behavioral therapies, including fluid management, can be added in order to increase your response to bladder retraining.

The central tenet of timed voiding and bladder retraining for urge incontinence requires that you go to the toilet before the urge to urinate can strike. For example, if you are planning to go shopping, you should try to use the toilet before leaving your house and then try again as soon as you reach the store or the mall, rather than waiting. Once you get the idea, you can just let common sense be your guide. Over the course of time, you can bladder "train" yourself to be completely dry.

How well does bladder retraining work? In a 1991 study at the Medical College of Virginia, one hundred healthy women over the age of fifty-five participated in a bladder retraining program. Of this group, 12 percent were completely cured, while 75 percent experienced significant improvement. The women in this group had stress, urge, and mixed incontinence. These results are extremely encouraging.

PELVIC FLOOR EXERCISES, OR KEGELS

Pelvic floor exercises, or Kegels, are simple exercises that you can do by yourself at any time. You can also do them just about anywhere, because no one will know you are doing them.

If done correctly and consistently, these exercises are very effective for stress, urge, and mixed urinary incontinence. These exercises strengthen your pelvic floor muscles, making it less likely that urine will leak out as a result of a weakened sphincter muscle, treating stress urinary incontinence. They are also effective in shutting off unwanted bladder contractions, thus treating urge incontinence.

Pelvic floor muscles are located under the bladder and urethra; in women, they help to hold the bladder, urethra, uterus, vagina, and rectum in place. Normally, strong pelvic floor muscles keep the urethra closed to prevent the leakage of urine. Then, when you are on the toilet and want to urinate, the pelvic floor muscles relax, allowing urine to pass out of the bladder.

As you know, one of the major causes of stress incontinence is weak pelvic floor muscles that are unable to hold the urine in properly. Properly performed, Kegel exercises strengthen these muscles, preventing the loss of urine during the physical activity that causes stress urinary incontinence. It is important to do Kegel exercises every day in order to maximize their effect and optimally strength the pelvic floor. In addition to the long-term benefits of Kegel exercises, immediate results can be seen if you can readily identify those activities which predictably result in stress incontinence. In these instances, a simultaneous and sustained Kegel exercise can prevent the leakage of urine. For example, if you know that you leak during a cough, then you should train yourself to do a pelvic floor exercise at the instant you feel a cough coming on. The properly performed Kegel will prevent the squirt of urine during the cough.

On the other hand, in patients with urge urinary incontinence, a properly performed Kegel exercise will shut off an unwanted involuntary bladder contraction if done correctly. It is well known that repeated quick forceful contractions of the pelvic floor will inhibit bladder activity. Therefore, if you suffer from urgency and urge urinary incontinence, you can be taught to do a series of Kegel exercises at the first sign of urinary urgency. This will eliminate the sense of urgency and prevent urinary leakage from occurring. Of course, if you suffer from urge urinary incontinence, it is also necessary to do regular pelvic floor exercises so you gain the awareness and strength necessary to properly shut off the unwanted involuntary bladder contraction when you need to.

If you are are healthy and have no problems with urinary leakage, doing regular Kegels may prevent incontinence from ever developing. If you are already incontinent to some degree, Kegels can improve your condition and may, in some cases, even cure it altogether. No matter what the state of your urinary system, you will almost certainly benefit from doing regular Kegels.

How Kegels Got Their Name

Kegel exercises are named after Arnold Kegel, M.D., a Los Angeles gynecologist who described them in 1948. In an article in the American Journal of Obstetrics and Gynecology entitled "Progressive Resistance Exercise in the Functional Restoration of the Perineal Muscles," Dr. Kegel described the exercises as a good treatment option for women suffering from stress incontinence. He pointed out that many women are not even aware that these muscles exist and he suggested that after a woman is instructed in how to tighten and draw them up, her doctor should examine her to make sure she is doing the contractions properly.

How to Do Kegels

Although Kegels are simple to do, you may have problems finding or identifying the right muscles. That's why it is a good idea to check with your doctor to be certain you are doing them correctly. Many women with persistent urinary incontinence believe that they are doing Kegel exercises correctly or thought that they were doing them correctly when they were not. This has led to much frustration and subsequently to the misguided belief by some patients and doctors alike that Kegel exercises don't work. Many scientific studies have shown, however, that Kegel exercises, when done correctly and consistently, are quite effective in treating urinary incontinence. Before giving up on pelvic floor exercises as ineffective treatment, even if you have tried them before, make sure that you are doing them correctly. Be checked by your doctor while doing Kegel exercises to ensure that you are doing them properly. Your doctor may also have a booklet with illustrations on how to do pelvic floor exercises. Often, however, a booklet or simple verbal instructions are not enough. If pelvic floor exercises have not been effective in treating your incontinence, you should be checked physically by your doctor to ensure that you are doing them correctly.

Here are the steps you can follow for learning to do these exercises correctly (information on many of the aids discussed is found later in this chapter):

Find the correct muscles: While you are urinating, try to stop the flow. Then start and stop the flow a few times. When you do this, you are tightening and relaxing your pelvic floor muscles.

When you try to stop the flow of urine, you will also get an idea of how strong your pelvic floor muscles are. If you can stop the flow instantaneously and easily and can do it several times, your muscles are probably working well; if you have trouble, your muscles are weak and need strengthening.

Pelvic floor muscles are also the same muscles that you tighten in order to stop yourself from passing gas, so you can use this fact as a way to find them.

Finally, you can locate these muscles by putting a finger inside your vagina and squeezing in the same way you would if you were trying to stop the flow of urine. The muscles that you feel tightening around your finger are your pelvic floor muscles.

After you locate the correct muscles, you should *not* exercise them every day *while* you are urinating. You may want to test the strength of your pelvic floor muscles and check your progress once every few weeks by seeing how well you can stop the flow of urine, but you should not do this on a daily basis.

Why? The reason is that if you repeat any behavior often enough, you can end up teaching yourself bad habits, even without meaning to. In the long run, it is not healthy for you to stop the natural flow of urine because you can end up trying to urinate with a closed or partially closed urethra—definitely not a good idea! That can cause your urine to back up and if carried to an extreme, it could even result in infections and damage to your kidneys.

Tighten your pelvic floor muscles: When you are certain you have located the correct muscles, begin to practice when you are not urinating. Tighten your pelvic floor muscles, pulling them in and also up, and hold them for five to ten seconds; then relax them for five to ten seconds. Do this for five or ten minutes at a time several times a day. You should *not* tighten your abdominal or buttock muscles when you do pelvic floor exercises. If you are unable to isolate your pelvic floor muscles from the abdomen or buttock muscles, then you are not doing them correctly. It is important to contract *only* the pelvic floor muscles when doing pelvic floor exercises. If you are unable to contract the pelvic floor muscles in isolation, then you may need an adjunctive training aid, such as biofeedback, to help you learn.

Don't be concerned if you are unable to hold the muscles tight for a full five to ten seconds when you first begin. Simply hold them tight for as long as you can and if it is only one or two seconds, let go and immediately tighten them again. As you practice, your ability to hold them longer will improve and the time interval will increase.

Again, when you tighten your pelvic floor muscles, make sure that you do not also tighten other parts of your body, such as your abdomen or buttocks. As you do the exercises, you should also not be moving any part of your body, such as your buttocks, thighs, or stomach. Only the pelvic floor muscles should be in motion, tightening and relaxing.

Increase number of contractions gradually: Ask your doctor how many times you should exercise your pelvic floor muscles at a single session and how many sessions you should perform each day. Many women benefit from doing the exercises three to five times a day with about fifteen contractions each time, while others may do the exercises every hour or perform as many as thirty-five or forty contractions each time.

It is generally recommended that you do the pelvic floor exercises often, but most importantly, remember to do them. For example, most people eat three meals per day, so a reasonable therapeutic regimen might be to do Kegel exercises thirty to thirty-five times at each meal. By associating these exercises with an activity that you do every day, it is easier to remember to do them. However, experts vary on the ideal frequency and number of daily contractions, with recommendations ranging from between thirty to three hundred contractions per day, so it is best to ask your doctor what frequency and number of total daily contractions are best for you.

Integrate Kegel exercises into your daily routine: You can do Kegels almost any time, especially when you are sitting and watching television, reading, driving, or talking on the phone. You can also do them while you are lying down or while you are standing. You can do them in the office or during dinner and no one will know because if you are doing them properly, your body will not be moving.

If you have stress incontinence, you should do Kegels when you cough, laugh, sneeze, exercise, lift heavy items, or at any other times when an increase in abdominal pressure may cause urinary leakage or has caused you leakage in the past.

If you suffer from urge incontinence, another obvious time to use Kegels is when you feel that you may be about to leak urine. By doing these exercises, you should be able to hold back the urine until the urgency resolves. In this way, Kegels can also be useful.

Use vaginal weights or cones: One way you may increase the effectiveness of your pelvic floor exercises is by doing them with vaginal weights or cones placed in your vagina. These devices, which come in different weights, are usually held in the vagina twice a day for fifteen minutes each time. When the weights are in place, the pelvic floor muscles must be contracted around them to hold them in, strengthening these muscles. As pelvic floor muscles strengthen over time, you can begin to use heavier weights.

Use biofeedback and electrical stimulation: Biofeedback can also help you to find out if you are exercising the correct muscles. Electrical stimulation can help develop your pelvic floor muscles, doing the Kegel exercises for you while you relax.

Be patient: There is no hard and fast rule about how long it takes to see a difference in the strength of your pelvic floor muscles, but most women experience noticeable results in two or three months. Be patient and keep working at it. Even if you don't notice a significant improvement, keep doing them, since they will eventually strengthen your pelvic floor muscles and can not harm you in any way.

Set a schedule: Because you want to remember to do the Kegels on a regular basis, it is a good idea to set a daily schedule with reminders. You may decide you want to do them during meals, on the way to work, or when you wake up and before you go to sleep. You could do them when you read the daily paper or watch the evening news. Some women leave themselves notes as reminders or write them on their daily schedules.

Combine Kegels with other therapies: Doing Kegels to strengthen your pelvic floor muscles and prevent or improve incontinence is beneficial because it doesn't cost anything, it can be done any time, there are no side effects, and most importantly, it can be successfully combined with many other incontinence therapies for maximum effectiveness.

The Results of Kegels

Studies have shown that Kegels usually improve your condition when you suffer from mild to moderate stress incontinence. Of course, in order to be effective, you must do these exercises on a regular basis. Doing them every now and then, when you happen to think of them, is not enough to make any real difference.

According to these studies, Kegel exercises improve stress incontinence for between 30 and 70 percent of the women who do them, and they cure the condition in about 20 percent of these women. They are especially effective for mild stress incontinence, where there is not frequent or significant urinary leakage. In addition, it may take as long as three months for any improvement to be evident, so you should not get discouraged if you fail to see results right away or even in the first few weeks you are doing the exercises. Be patient and do not give up!

Of course, there are some women who do not show any positive results from doing Kegels, but in some cases, that is because they are not exercising the correct muscles or are not doing the exercises in the proper way. You must be absolutely certain that you are exercising the correct muscles and doing the contractions properly. That is why it is so important to obtain instructions and periodic monitoring from your physician. In fact, one Canadian urogynecologist estimated that at least 60 percent of women doing Kegel exercises do not perform them correctly.

It's also important for you to realize that you have to perform the Kegel exercises for the rest of your life if you want to maintain your improvement. If you stop doing them, your pelvic floor muscles can weaken and your incontinence may return or get worse. You should remember that other than during sexual activity and urination or defecation, your pelvic floor muscles do not normally get any exercise and by doing Kegels on your own, you will be keeping them in good working order.

In addition to helping you overcome stress incontinence, Kegel exercises have an added benefit: by tightening pelvic floor muscles in your vaginal area, they can also increase your sexual pleasure. Many women are surprised and delighted by this unexpected side effect, and quite a few women report that after practicing Kegels, they experienced either their first orgasms or orgasms that were greatly improved.

Biofeedback

By using biofeedback, you can learn to identify your pelvic floor muscles and master the proper techniques for exercising and strengthening them. Biofeedback technology has been around for many years and was, for a time, considered an alternative therapy. In recent years, it has gained legitimacy and is now widely accepted for the treatment of a number of medical disorders, including urinary incontinence.

With certain types of biofeedback, you are attached to electrodes which electronically monitor your body functions, including your heartbeat, brain waves, and muscle contractions. By observing the monitor and seeing how these functions change, you can learn to make changes in your own body in order to achieve the desired results.

Biofeedback is helpful if you have either stress or urge incontinence.

You have just seen that one of the most effective behavioral techniques is pelvic floor muscle exercise (or Kegels), and biofeedback can help you to monitor your progress as you work to strengthen your pelvic floor muscles by practicing these exercises.

In order to monitor your pelvic floor muscles using biofeedback, small monitors are inserted near or in your vagina or rectum and, as you perform the exercises to contract your pelvic floor muscles, you can follow your progress on the screen and see how well you are doing. The monitor also helps you if you are uncertain about whether or not you are exercising the correct muscles when you perform the Kegels. Finally, biofeedback allows you to take control of your problem and be pro-active in seeking a remedy.

Although there are more biofeedback centers today than in the past, it may still be difficult for you to find one, especially outside of major cities. In addition, this therapy is not always covered by insurance.

If your insurance company will not cover this therapy, you can sometimes have your doctor appeal to them in writing, although that is not always successful. Sometimes, an insurance company will pay for biofeedback if it is performed by a licensed physical therapist, which must be prescribed by your physician.

VAGINAL WEIGHTS OR CONES

As you just learned, vaginal weights or cones are devices that give you another method for strengthening your pelvic floor muscles. You simply place the weighted cone-shaped inserts in your vagina twice a day and keep them in place for about fifteen minutes each time. In order to hold the cones in place, you must contract your pelvic floor muscles.

Vaginal cones come in different weights and when you begin using them, you start with a lower weight. As your pelvic floor muscles strengthen, you will be given heavier cones, which require greater muscle strength to hold in place.

In this way, you will gradually develop more and more control of your pelvic floor muscles, increasing your bladder control. Studies comparing the effectiveness of Kegels with the use of these devices show that the vaginal cones appear to be effective, and using them makes your pelvic floor muscle-strengthening techniques much easier to learn.

ELECTRICAL STIMULATION

Electrical stimulation is a technique that allows you to practice pelvic floor exercises in your own home with the assistance of an electrical device. This machine uses a sensor insert or probe, which is placed into your vagina or rectum and directly stimulates your pelvic floor muscles. In essence, the stimulator produces a "Kegel exercise" without you having to do anything.

Using this machine takes away the worry that you are not exercising the correct muscles. Without any real effort on your part, the pelvic electrical stimulator gradually strengthens and tightens your pelvic floor muscles and also retrains the nerves that control your bladder function.

Electrical stimulation may be useful in both stress and urge incontinence and is especially effective when done with the supervision of a doctor, since that will usually motivate you to use it on a regular basis. However, these stimulators can be expensive and they are not covered by all insurance policies.

The Neocontrol Device

This patented device, made by Neotonus of Marietta, Georgia, is being studied for use in the treatment of stress, urge, and mixed incontinence. A non-invasive therapy, the Neocontrol uses a new technology called *Extracorporeal Magnetic Innervation.*

The device creates highly focused pulsing magnetic fields which course through a chair located above the machine. As you sit in the chair, fully clothed, the magnetic fields pulsate, exercising your pelvic floor muscles and causing them to contract and relax.

Treatment with this device is by prescription only. Sessions are usually half an hour in length and the usual course of treatment is twice a week for eight weeks. Some excellent results have been reported with this chair, and additional studies are ongoing to fully understand its effectiveness in treating stress incontinence, urge incontinence, and pelvic pain.

Once again, with this device, the benefits of Kegels may be achieved with less effort or chance for error than if you do them on your own. But this therapy is also costly and is not covered by all insurance plans.

12

ACUPUNCTURE

With the growing popularity of the alternative health movement, more and more traditionally trained physicians are learning about different therapies that may be useful for treating incontinence. Some of these approaches have been around for a long time. Acupuncture is one of these therapies.

In use for over a thousand years as part of the ancient system of medical care in China, acupuncture has enjoyed great popularity in the United States in recent years. Acupuncture is used to treat a very wide range of physical and mental disorders and has attracted the attention of many physicians who have either learned the technique themselves or referred people to trained acupuncturists.

Arising from the idea that life is based on a free flow of energy and disease results when energy is blocked, acupuncture uses tiny, thin needles placed on specific points along the body's nerve pathways (meridians) in order to restore natural energy and allow the body to heal itself.

Acupuncturists believe that the source of incontinence problems lies in the urinary system, specifically in the kidneys and bladder. Treatment does not focus on these organs alone, however, but on restoring the flow of energy throughout the entire body.

In traditional acupuncture, the practitioner examines the tongue and wrist pulses in order to diagnose a disorder. Then, he or she inserts needles at specific meridians, attempting to restore the proper flow of energy.

In modern acupuncture, the practitioner diagnoses a disorder through a more traditional physical examination, much like a Western-trained doctor would perform. Treatment usually involves fewer needles and the practitioner leaves them in for a shorter period of time than with the traditional form.

Women who try acupuncture for incontinence sometimes see results after only one session, while others need up to twelve sessions of half hour or an hour. Of course, there are also many women who do not respond to acupuncture at all. In fact, there are few, if any, studies that have scientifically evaluated the value of acupuncture for stress or urge incontinence. This treatment has also been reported as occasionally effective for women suffering from the pain and discomfort of interstitial cystitis.

If you want to try acupuncture, you should discuss it with your doctor and ask for a referral. If your doctor is unable to give you the name of an acupuncture practitioner, you can ask friends or healthcare professionals who are familiar with this type of therapy, or you can contact: The American Academy of Medical Acupuncture (see Appendix A for contact information).

They can provide you with a referral to an acupunturist in your area. Always be certain that the practitioner you choose has proper training and a state license if one is required where you live. You should also find out if the acupuncturist has experience treating urinary incontinence.

13

MEDICATION

One of the most common ways of treating incontinence is through prescription medication. Treatments include the use of drugs for different types of incontinence, as well as estrogen replacement. Using these medications can provide a fairly easy solution for many women.

ESTROGEN REPLACEMENT

Supplemental estrogen for postmenopausal women remains controversial. Some studies show benefits and others are inconclusive or indicate potential health problems. Some studies show that women on certain types of hormone replacement therapy (HRT) have lower risks of some kinds of cancer, but increased risk of strokes. Studies on the effects of HRT on the risk of some types of breast cancer remain inconclusive.

The estrogen used for treating incontinence is not exactly the same as the estrogen used for post-menopause. In some cases, it is in a far lower dose and is delivered in a topical cream or patch, rather than in a pill.

After menopause, the dramatic drop in levels of the female hormone estrogen may bring about vaginal dryness and a thinning of the tissues in the vagina and urinary tract. These events can cause a loss of muscle tone and elasticity, resulting in urinary incontinence.

Doctors have found that applying a low-dose estrogen cream to your vaginal area can effectively deliver the hormone directly to the urinary system to treat incontinence. In some cases, an estrogen ring (Estring), a plastic ring containing estrogen, is inserted into the vagina and replaced every three months. Because of its shape, it does not interfere with menstruation or with sexual activity.

Another recent development for localized estrogen replacement is Vagifem. This is a tiny estrogen impregnated pellet which is placed into the vagina once or twice weekly using a special applicator. It releases estrogens directly to the vagina and nearby urinary tract.

Studies of the use of low-dose estrogen for incontinence are mixed. Some show that stress incontinence improves with estrogen supplementation; other studies show that only urge incontinence (and not stress incontinence) improves, and still other studies showing little or no improvement in either type, especially over the long term. Because these studies are so inconclusive, the decision about whether or not to use estrogen to treat incontinence is not an easy one for you and your doctor to make.

If you use HRT for the symptoms of menopause, one important factor to remember is that there is a chance that you will experience some troublesome side effects. It is also possible that if you use the lower-dose topical estrogen creams or patches for incontinence, you may experience some of these side effects. They can include weight gain, tenderness in your breasts, nausea, hot flashes, cramps, headaches, and dizziness. Of course, these side effects are less likely when a low dose is used, but they are still possibilities that you will want to take into consideration.

Estrogen can sometimes be used if you have stress incontinence or urge incontinence. Depending on your individual case, the use of estrogen may be a good option for you.

Deciding whether or not to use estrogen is a complex decision that you need to make in consultation with your physician. You will have to weigh all the potential pros and cons, taking the specific details of your medical history and incontinence into consideration before you can decide whether or not you want to try it. It is important for you to discuss this thoroughly with your doctor before making your decision.

Types of Medication for Incontinence

Many different types of medication are used to treat incontinence. These drugs either relax the bladder, if it is overactive, as it is with urge incontinence; or tighten the sphincter muscle, if it is weak, as it is with stress incontinence. They include the following:

Anticholinergic Medications

These include tolterodine tartrate (Detrol LA) and oxybutynin chloride (Ditropan XL), the most commonly prescribed anticholinergic medications, they are used primarily for urge incontinence. These drugs are effective in treating urge incontinence because they relax the detrusor muscle but do not relax the outlet to the bladder. In other words, they counteract the spasms of the overactive bladder that are causing urgency and leakage, thereby allowing more urine to be held in your bladder.

However, these drugs do not increase the warning time that you need in order to get to the bathroom in time once you get that strong urge to go. That is why it is essential to combine them with behavioral therapy, such as timed voiding, which can improve that part of the problem. Although these drugs are often well tolerated, you may be bothered by such unpleasant side effects as dry mouth, headache, constipation, blurred vision, indigestion, and dry eyes. In some cases, the side effects are bad enough to cause you to discontinue using the medication. Notably, although these drugs seem to work equally well in controlling overactive bladder symptoms and urge incontinence, it seems from recent studies that the unpleasant side effects resulting from the use of anticholinergic drugs is much less severe with Detrol LA than the other available agents.

Overall, these medications are effective, with studies indicating that the number of incontinence incidents due to overactive bladder decline between 40 and 70 percent with the use of these drugs.

Alpha-Adrenergic Agonists

These are found in over-the counter decongestants, cold medications, and appetite suppressants including ephedrine and pseudoephedrine (Sudafed), which have occasionally been helpful in the treatment of stress incontinence, especially when combined with estrogen. They act to increase muscle tone and tighten the bladder neck and urethra, helping to better hold urine in the bladder.

You should note that phenylpropanolamine (PPA), an alpha-adrenergic agonist, has recently come under fire for its potentially dangerous side effects, including stroke, rapid heartbeat, and anxiety. It is in the process of being withdrawn, so it is no longer recommended.

Tricyclic Antidepressants

Tricyclicantidepressants, such as imipramine (Tofranil), may be used to treat both stress incontinence and urge incontinence, because they have effects on both the urethra and the bladder. These drugs calm an overactive bladder and are sometimes combined with anticholinergics, a drug class which has similar effects. However, because of the possibility of unwanted side effects and the possibility of problems when combined with other medications, if you use these drugs, you must be very carefully monitored by your doctor.

Other Drugs

Antibiotics may be used to treat urinary tract infections that are associated with incontinence. Other drugs which may be used to treat *urge incontinence* include the following: Bentyl, Cystospaz, Cystospaz-M, Levsin, Prelief, Pro-Banthine, Urised and Urispas. Other drugs which have been used to treat *stress incontinence* include Ornade, Entex, Entex-LA, and Sudafed.

USING MEDICATION

If you decide to use medication for your condition, remember to:

- Take your medication exactly as prescribed by your doctor.
- Ask about the potential side effects of the medication.
- Immediately report any side effects to your doctor.
- Find out how long it takes for improvements to occur and be patient.
- Make sure your doctor knows about any other medications you use.
- Ask your doctor if another medication might be better if you feel the drug is not effective or the side effects bother you.

You should be aware that medication does not help everyone, but it can be an important part of a program to provide assistance, to combine with other therapies, or to improve conditions that do not respond to other treatments.

WHICH MEDICATIONS FOR WHICH PROBLEM?

Some medications are useful for stress incontinence, some for urge incontinence, and some for both. To summarize:

For Urge Incontinence:

- Anticholinergics
- Tricyclic antidepressants (sometimes)
- Estrogen (sometimes)

In general, drugs for urge incontinence are much more effective than those for stress incontinence.

For Stress Incontinence

- Alpha-adrenergic agonists
- Tricyclic antidepressants (sometimes)
- Estrogen (sometimes)

For urinary tract infections

- Antibiotics
- Antibacterial agents

HOW LONG DO THE DRUGS TAKE TO WORK?

You may wonder how long you should wait before seeing positive results from your medication. Unfortunately, there is no hard and fast rule. Your results will vary according to the type of medication you use, the severity of your condition, and how your body responds to the drug. It can take anywhere from a couple of days or weeks, to a couple of months for you to see good results.

If you find that the medication has not done its job after three months, it is unlikely that it will have any positive effect on you. At that point, you will want to ask your doctor for a change in medication or a change in the dose of your medication, either of which could bring you some improvement.

14

CHOOSING SURGERY

As you are now aware, surgery is usually, although not always, the treatment of last resort for urinary incontinence. In general, it is used when all the other, less invasive treatments do not provide satisfactory results. However, if your condition is really severe or caused by structural problems that can be surgically corrected, surgery may be your first, best, or only option.

It's also possible that you do not want to be bothered with less invasive treatments, even when they might help. If all you want is for your leakage problem to be fixed as quickly as possible, you may tell your doctor that you want to proceed immediately. If a surgical procedure is a good option for you, your doctor and you may decide to proceed with surgery as an initial treatment. When surgery is appropriate:

- Other, less invasive treatments have not worked.
- You have severe incontinence and other treatments will not help.
- You want to have surgery to improve or cure your condition as quickly as possible.

FACTORS INVOLVED IN YOUR DECISION

Your decision about whether or not to undergo a surgical procedure to treat your incontinence is complicated and you should not make it lightly. You should think about it very carefully while you take a lot of different factors into consideration, including:

- The specific cause or causes of your condition
- The impact your condition has on your life
- How willing you are to try other methods of treatment first
- How long you are willing to wait to get results
- How you feel about surgery in general
- Whether you are prepared to be hospitalized and away from your regular activities while you take time to recover
- How confident you are in your surgeon
- Whether you feel that surgery is the best, or the only, option for treating your condition

No one can make this decision for you, but if you think things through and thoroughly discuss all the important factors with your physician, and with your partner, close friends, and relatives, you will be able to make an informed decision about whether surgery is your best option.

SURGICAL PROS AND CONS

Surgical procedures can range from injections in your doctor's office to very complex operations that take hours to perform in the operating room. In most cases, if you have surgery it will involve hospitalization and recovery time. It can also be expensive and it always has some risk of adverse side effects. In certain cases, surgery may not cure your incontinence completely and you may still require other treatments.

Even so, there are a number of surgical procedures for stress and urge incontinence that are extremely effective and help many women to overcome or vastly improve their bladder control problems. While the other treatments that have been discussed are usually helpful, making surgery unnecessary, it is still important for you to understand surgical procedures and find out if they may be an option to help your specific condition. You should also be aware that surgery for stress incontinence is far more common than surgery for urge incontinence. In fact, surgery for urge incontinence is performed quite rarely.

Some surgical procedures for incontinence require a hospital stay of one to three days, although there are some newer procedures that do not require you to stay in the hospital overnight. Recovery periods vary according to the procedure and the individual, but they usually range from one or two days to up to six or eight weeks.

SURGERY FOR STRESS URINARY INCONTINENCE

Well over one hundred different operations have been developed for the treatment of stress incontinence. The choice of procedure depends on a number of factors, including:

- Experience of the surgeon
- Availability and effectiveness of the procedure
- Invasiveness, risks, and possible adverse outcomes of the surgery
- Recovery and convalescence time
- Coexistent problems that might be handled surgically at the same time as your incontinence problem
- The underlying anatomical and physiological problems which have caused your incontinence

Problems that can be handled by surgery include:

- Pelvic organ prolapse (bladder [cystocele], urethra)

- Very weak sphincter or pelvic floor muscles
- Fistulas
- Congenital problems/birth defects

Some of the major surgical procedures described below create support for the fallen bladder or urethra, securing them in their proper places, while others provide support and directly compress the urethra and sphincter muscles, so that coughing, exercising, or performing other daily routine activities no longer cause urine leakage. Before we look at major surgery, let's examine the use of collagen injections, which can be very helpful in treating stress incontinence.

Periurethral Injectable Agents: Collagen

Urine leakage due to a faulty urethra and weak sphincter muscle can be treated with collagen injections directly into the urethral tissue, near the neck of the bladder. The injected collagen tends to bulk up and swell these tissues, closing off the bladder neck and making it better able to contain urine in the bladder.

If you have stress incontinence and have had previous surgery that was not entirely successful, there is a very good chance you will be helped by collagen injections. Or if you have stress incontinence and do not want to have major surgery, you may also be a good candidate for collagen. Collagen is a naturally occurring material that seems to have few side effects. However, collagen does tend to get absorbed into your body over time, so the injections must sometimes be repeated in order to maintain a good effect.

Although the injections can be performed under general anesthesia or spinal anesthesia, sometimes just a local anesthetic in the urethra is used for the injections, which are performed in your doctor's office. The procedure takes about twenty minutes. Function is sometimes restored after only one injection, but some patients may need a series of injections, which are usually performed several weeks or months apart.

One study showed that approximately eighty percent of women using collagen injections for incontinence were either improved or cured after a series of three injections. The advantages of collagen injections are that they are relatively quick, minimally invasive, and, for the most part, pain-free. Another advantage is that the recovery or convalescence time is very brief (just one day).

Collagen injections are rather expensive, so that could be a potential drawback. However, they are covered by most insurance plans, including Medicare. Another drawback is the fact that some women may be allergic to the collagen material, which is usually derived from cows. Because of this allergic response, a skin test is performed several weeks prior to injection as a precaution.

Side effects include a burning sensation after urination, a little blood in the urine or a urinary tract infection, but these are not too common and usually clear up on their own after a short time.

You should also be aware that instead of collagen, other materials, including Teflon and fat, are sometimes used for similar purposes.

Your decision about whether or not to use collagen or similar injections for your condition is one that you should discuss very carefully with your physician.

Advantages:

- Minimally invasive
- Sometimes performed in the doctor's office
- Procedure takes only twenty minutes
- Studies show up to eighty percent improvement or cure after three injections
- No pain
- One-day recovery period

Disadvantages:

- Expensive if not covered by insurance
- May require repeated injections for successful treatment
- Possible allergies to collagen

Abdominal Operations

Abdominal operations for repairing stress incontinence were considered the "gold standard" treatment for a long time. Many surgeons were trained using these techniques and still do primarily these types of operations. There are many types of abdominal operations, but the most popular are the Burch Colpo suspension and the Marshall-Marchetti-Krantz vesicourethropexy.

All of the abdominal operations are done through a long incision in the abdominal wall, usually about five to six inches in length. Using stitches in the tissues adjacent to the bladder and urethra, these operations elevate or support the urethra and bladder neck.

The incision may be horizontal ("bikini line") or vertical, depending on the patient's preference. If there has been previous abdominal surgery, as with a hysterectomy, for example, the surgeon will usually try to use the same incision for this surgery.

Long-term success rates with these types of procedures are reported to be about 85 to 90 percent, but these rates may vary considerably among surgeons.

Advantages:

- The familiarity of the abdominal anatomy and surgical technique to most surgeons
- Durability (these operations have been done for over fifty years)
- The opportunity to repair coexistent abdominal problems through the same incision

Disadvantages:

- A large incision
- Prolonged hospital stay and recovery period
- Increased post-operative discomfort
- Potential side effects, including bleeding, infection, and damage to other abdominal contents

Abdominal Operations Using Laparoscopy

In some cases, a surgeon may use laparoscopic surgery, or "keyhole" surgery, to perform an abdominal operation. These operations use a thin, telescope-like instrument called a laparoscope to see into the abdomen and perform the surgery. This allows the surgeon to make the needed repairs using only a few small incisions in the abdomen (usually between one half and one inch-long). The method has not been in use long enough for long-term studies to have been completed regarding possible side effects or durability over time, so the quality and permanence of results are still uncertain. Even though laparoscopic techniques have been in use for close to a hundred years, they have only been used for abdominal operations to treat stress incontinence for the past few years.

Advantages:

• Short hospitalization, often only one day
• Less invasive than traditional surgery

Disadvantages:

• Potential side effects, including bleeding, infection and damage to other abdominal contents

• Long-term results still not known

Vaginal Operations

Alternatives to the abdominal operations for stress incontinence are procedures performed through small incisions in the vagina. These operations are categorized as either transvaginal "needle" suspensions (because a small needle carrier is used during the operation to carry the stitches from the vaginal incisions to the abdomen) or slings, which create a permanent hammock-like support for the bladder neck and urethra. These techniques are a minimally invasive alternative to the abdominal procedures.

Advantages:

- Avoiding a large, painful abdominal incision
- Shorter operative time
- Less post-operative discomfort
- Shorter hospital stay and convalescence

Disadvantages:

- A technically demanding surgery
- Greater risk of injury to the bladder and urethra during passage of the needles during the surgery
- A potentially greater risk of bleeding and, for the "needle" suspensions (but not the slings), a lower long-term cure rate

NEEDLE SUSPENSIONS

In 1959, the original transvaginal needle suspension was described, using stainless steel wires for support. Many modifications of this original procedure have been made since that time. The common feature with all of these procedures is that the abdominal wall muscles are not incised and the stitches are placed through small incisions in the vagina.

Similar to the abdominal procedures, the stitches are placed into the tissues adjacent to the bladder and urethra, but since they are put in through small incisions in the vagina, they must be carried up through the abdomen somewhat blindly, or without direct visualization by the surgeon. This is done with a specialized instrument, called a needle carrier. The stitches are then tied to the muscular abdominal wall through tiny incisions in the skin.

Sometimes, the stitches are secured to the pelvic bones instead of the muscle, using special devices called bone anchors. Many surgeons are not familiar with these techniques and are not prepared to do these types of operations.

There are several types of these procedures, each differing with regard to the specific type of stitches used, the type of vaginal incision, and the extent of surgery in the vagina. Long-term success rates for the vaginal needle suspensions are about 65 to 75 percent, but like the abdominal operations, the success rates vary considerably among surgeons.

SLINGS

Slings are performed through types of incisions similar to the needle suspensions. However, instead of using stitches to suspend the tissues next to the bladder and urethra up to the abdominal wall, a sling procedure involves placing a tough, long-lasting material underneath the urethra, like a hammock, and then taping or stitching this material to the abdominal muscles or pubic bone.

Originally described almost 100 years ago, slings of various types have had a resurgence in popularity over the past several years. This may be a result of several factors, including a change in surgical approach due to the disappointing long-term durability of the needle suspensions, a better understanding of the causes of stress incontinence, and improvements in the operative technique of slings.

For many years, slings were only performed as a last ditch effort for women who had failed with other surgeries. That was because the operation was technically demanding and associated with a high rate of complications. Even so, the operation was highly successful and durable.

However, as modern operative techniques have evolved, slings have become easier and safer, although many surgeons still prefer not to do these operations. Usually, the slings used are made of fascia, the shiny, silver, leather-like covering of many of the muscles of the body.

The fascia is "harvested" from an incision in the abdomen (rectus abdominis fascia), or less commonly, the thigh (fascia lata) during the sling operation. Another source of fascia is from organ donors (cadaver fascia). This source of fascia is available commercially or from local hospital tissue banks.

Other slings are made from artificial material such as nylon, polypropylene, or Gortex. There are advantages and disadvantages to each type of sling material and it is best for you to discuss these pros and cons with your surgeon. The long-term success rates from the sling approach is 90 to 95 percent, and it is now probably considered the gold standard surgery for the treatment of stress urinary incontinence.

Tension-Free Vaginal Tape (TVT)

A relatively new procedure, tension-free vaginal tape (TVT), involves two very small incisions made in the abdomen and one in the vagina. This operation is done very quickly and the recovery time is quite brief. In some cases, it can be done with minimal anesthesia.

Instead of implanting a sling made of tissue, the surgeon uses a specialized instrument to place a type of mesh tape underneath the urethra to support it. Then, over time, tissue in the body grows through the mesh.

Used for stress incontinence, this procedure has not been around for many years. If it is of interest to you, discuss it with your doctor.

Advantages:

• Minimally invasive
• Requires only minimal anesthesia in some people
• Takes about half an hour to perform

Disadvantages:

• May not be available in every area
• Long-term results are not yet available

Anterior Repair

Anterior repair procedures can also be considered vaginal operations because they are performed entirely through the vagina. In this procedure, the surgeon takes tissue from both sides of the urethra and stitches them together under the urethra to create support.

Most anterior repair operations are done as part of another surgical procedure, such as a hysterectomy, rather than performed on their own. If you are having a hysterectomy or some other pelvic surgery, and are also incontinent, you might want to talk to your surgeon about the possibility of having this procedure.

Advantages:

- Takes only a short time to perform
- Can be helpful for some women

Disadvantages:

- Usually performed as part of other surgical procedures
- Long-term success rate, about 40 percent, is not as high as some other surgical procedures

ARTIFICIAL URINARY SPHINCTER IMPLANT

Surgeons can also implant an artificial urinary sphincter device if the sphincter is too damaged to repair and if the stress incontinence can not be helped with other approaches. The artificial urinary sphincter device is a complex, expensive, and somewhat involved intervention that is rarely performed for women with stress incontinence in the United States, but is more commonly used in Europe.

Advantages

- An option for women with seriously damaged urinary sphincters
- Results can be excellent with experienced surgeons

Disadvantages

- Most surgeons are not trained in implanting the device in women.
- Expensive
- Complex operation

- Many patients may require a second operation after initial placement, due to mechanical malfunction of the device, erosion, infection, or lack of effectiveness.

Surgery for Urge Incontinence

Although not performed as often, surgery for urge incontinence can be successful. There are two major types of procedures: sacral neuromodulation and augmentation cystoplasty.

Sacral Neuromodulation

Sometimes, when other approaches with urge incontinence fail, you may be helped by the implantation of a small stimulator device, called the Interstim. The Interstim implant is about the size of a small pager and is placed into the buttock. A thin wire is then attached to the device and is placed next to the nerves that control bladder function.

The device then gives off low-level electrical signals to these nerves, which help to control the emptying of the bladder. The Interstim device can be reprogrammed externally, with a hand-held magnet. Using a highly specialized computer, the device can be adjusted and customized to individual needs. As a result, your bladder may be able to function more normally, with a reduction or elimination of urge incontinence due to bladder overactivity. This procedure is relatively new, and was approved for widespread use in 1997. The initial results with this therapy are very promising.

Fortunately, a simple outpatient test, called a PNE, can be conducted several days to weeks prior to the surgical procedure to determine whether the Interstim will be effective. Only those people who have a positive response to the PNE are potential candidates for the operation.

Advantages:

- Customized and adjusted to individual needs
- Short-term results are promising
- An option when other approaches fail

Disadvantages:

• Invasive implantation of electrical device
• Possible mechanical failure with need for removing device and repairing or implanting a second one
• Long-term results unknown

Augmentation or Enlargement Cystoplasty

Augmentation cystoplasty is a surgical procedure that enlarges your bladder, making it capable of holding a greater amount of urine. This type of surgery can benefit those who suffer from urge incontinence and who have a bladder that does not hold a normal amount of urine.

This can occur if the bladder is very small, overactive, or lacking in elasticity due to neurological problems, such as spinal cord injuries or multiple sclerosis; damage to organs during childbirth; or from cancer radiation therapy.

In augmentation cystoplasty, the surgeon most commonly uses a piece of intestine or bowel to make the bladder larger. This is a complicated and highly specialized surgery which often involves a large abdominal incision and a prolonged hospital stay and convalescence. Augmentation cystoplasty is not recommended if you are unable or unwilling to catheterize yourself (see Chapter Fifteen), or if you have kidney disease, bowel disease, or urethral disease. The operation does not always cure urge incontinence, but it is a highly effective treatment for those women who do not derive satisfaction from other types of therapy. Because of the nature and complexity of the surgery, augmentation cystoplasty is usually reserved for women in whom nothing else has worked for their urge incontinence.

Advantages:

• It can be effective when all other approaches to treating urge incontinence have failed.

Disadvantages

- Does not always cure urge incontinence
- Complicated and specialized surgery
- Large abdominal incision
- Long hospitalization and recovery period
- Potential need for self-catheterization after surgery
- Not appropriate for those with kidney disease, bowel disease, or urethral disease

Other Surgical Procedures

In some cases, urge incontinence may be due to vaginal prolapse, a condition where the pelvic organs sag into the vagina and then cause obstruction of the urinary flow and urge incontinence. Vaginal prolapse involving the bladder may also be associated with stress incontinence. By surgically sewing the prolapsed organs back in place, incontinence is often significantly improved or cured.

Surgery for vaginal prolapse may involve different types of repair.

CYSTOCELE

When the bladder sags into the vagina, it is called a cystocele. A bladder that is not in place can cause bladder overactivity and urinary obstruction, as well as stress incontinence. Surgery to repair a cystocele involves moving the bladder back into its proper position and using sutures to anchor it.

UTERINE PROLAPSE

A uterine prolapse occurs when the uterus sags into the vagina, sometimes falling beyond the vaginal opening. This can create problems for normal urination and also may cause incontinence. Surgical procedures to repair a prolapsed uterus include sewing the uterus back into its proper place, and performing a hysterectomy to remove the uterus.

RECTOCELE AND ENTEROCELE

When the rectum bulges into the vagina, it is called a rectocele; when the small intestine bulges into the vagina, it is called an enterocele. As with a cystocele, surgery involves moving the bulging organ back into its proper place and anchoring it with sutures.

VAGINAL VAULT PROLAPSE

A vaginal vault prolapse occurs when the top of the vagina falls in on itself and sags out of the vaginal opening. This only occurs following a hysterectomy. The surgical procedure involves moving the vagina back into its proper position and anchoring it with sutures.

CHOOSING A SURGEON

If you have discussed your condition thoroughly with your physician and have decided that surgery is a good option for you, it is important that you feel confident about the surgeon you have chosen to perform your procedure. If you need to choose a surgeon, you can follow the guidelines presented in Chapter Seven for finding the right doctor. If you are under the care of a trusted physician who is not a surgeon, ask that physician to recommend a couple so that you can choose the one you like best.

As with choosing any physician, it is important that you talk with potential surgeons before making your decision. It is imperative that you find out about the surgeon's experience in performing the procedure you need. Ask how you can expect to feel after the operation and what long-term results you can anticipate.

Here are some questions you may want to ask in order to get the information you need, in addition to those listed in Chapter Seven.

The Surgeon's Experience

• How long have you been doing this procedure?

- How many procedures of this type have you done?

All other things being equal, you should select a surgeon who has been doing the procedure for a long period of time and has performed many operations.

The Surgical Procedure:

- How long will I be in the hospital?
- What are the possible side effects from the operation (such as temporary or permanent urinary urgency and frequency, nausea, vaginal shortening)?
- What are the usual results in a case like mine?
- What percentage of women who have this procedure are completely cured?
- What are the chances of my incontinence being completely cured? Improved? Worsened?
- Is there a chance that I might need additional surgery in the future?

Answers to these questions will help you form realistic expectations about your surgery, as well as provide you with insight into the surgeon's experience and expertise with a specific surgical procedure.

After Your Surgery

- How long will full recovery take?
- When will I be able to go back to work or carry out my regular activities?
- When will I be able to resume sexual activity?
- Will I be able to engage in sports and other activities that now cause urinary leakage?
- What kind of follow-up visits will I need?
- If I'm not completely cured, what other options do I have?

Answers to these questions will help you prepare for every possible outcome from surgery, which will help you make decisions about your options, just in case you do not get the results you want. The answers to these questions will also give you insight into the doctor's experience and expertise.

Second Opinions

It is always a good idea to get a second, and possibly even a third opinion before you decide on surgery or select a surgeon. Most health plans will cover the cost of a second opinion. Don't be in a hurry. Chances are you have been coping with incontinence for a while, so another week or so won't hurt.

While you may want to have surgery immediately because you think it is the best option for curing or significantly improving your condition, it is usually wise to be cautious and choose surgery only when everything else has failed or has been determined not to be an appropriate treatment for you.

When you consult with different surgeons, be aware of whether options other than surgery are discussed. Always review the results of all your diagnostic tests with the surgeon and then ask if surgery is the best choice for you and if so, why.

It is important for you to feel comfortable about having surgery. If you feel that you are being pressured to have surgery, or if you are not convinced that it is the best or the first choice for you, get other opinions.

Preparing for Surgery

If you follow these suggestions, you may find that the surgical procedure will go more smoothly and your recovery may be quicker.

- Do not smoke. If you are a smoker, stop smoking at least two weeks before your operation. The primary reason is that smoking can increase your risk of complications from anesthesia because it increases mucus production in the lungs.
- Do not take aspirin, aspirin-like products (nonsteroidal anti-inflammatory prescription products, such as Vioxx and Celebrex), or over-the-counter ibuprofen (Advil or similar medications) for

one week prior to surgery. These products could increase bleeding during surgery.

- Ask your doctor if there are any medications, including over-the-counter drugs and vitamins, that you should avoid prior to surgery.
- Make sure you have had all the diagnostic tests that your surgeon requires.
- Arrange for someone to help you at home during your recovery period. Depending on your surgical procedure and how well you recover, you may not be able to lift heavy objects, climb stairs, lift, bend, drive, go to work, or do housework for anywhere from a few days to a few weeks.
- As a precaution, be sure to ask your doctor if there is anything else you should do to prepare for surgery.

POSSIBLE RISK FACTORS

Remember that every surgical procedure involves a risk. There is no such thing as an operation that is one hundred percent risk-free. Some of the risk factors for the surgical procedures for incontinence are:

- Pain (usually temporary and treated with medication)
- Urinary urgency and frequency is one of the most frequent side effects. It is often temporary, but there is always the possibility that it may be permanent.
- Infection
- Bleeding
- Nausea or vomiting
- Fever
- Burning sensation while urinating
- Inability to urinate (urinary retention), often only temporary, but sometimes permanent
- Blood clots in the legs and pelvis, that could travel to the lungs (pulmonary embolism)
- Damage to nerves, muscles, and nearby pelvic structures
- Complications from anesthesia

• Vaginal shortening or narrowing, causing sexual dysfunction or painful intercourse

After going through this list, you may well feel alarmed. You shouldn't; The fact is that most women experience only mild side effects and only on a temporary basis. The chances are very good that you will come through surgery with only a short recovery time.

THE RESULTS OF SURGERY

Studies of the effectiveness of surgery for urinary incontinence show a high rate of success and cure. A study done in the late 1990s by the American Urological Association found that surgery was so effective that it could be recommended as a first treatment for people with severe incontinence whose condition seriously interfered with their daily lives.

Analyzing 282 studies of four basic surgical procedures used at that time (retropubic suspension, transvaginal needle suspension, the pubovaginal sling and anterior repair), the analysis found that abdominal operations and sling procedures had the highest cure rates, while transvaginal suspensions and anterior repairs had lower cure rates. The actual results of your surgery will depend on many factors, including your general health, the severity of your incontinence, the type of surgery you choose, and the expertise of your surgeon.

15

HELPFUL PRODUCTS AND DEVICES

There are treatments for incontinence that do not fall into the categories of behavioral techniques, drug therapy, or surgery, including a variety of anti-incontinence devices and other products which have recently come on the market. It is possible that, either temporarily or on a long-term basis, you may want some of these incontinence products to help you manage your condition.

Be aware that the manufacturers of these items are constantly changing or refining them, and also bringing new ones on the market. By the time you read this book, some of the products described here may no longer be available and others may have replaced them. That is why it is so important to keep up with the latest products so you will have access to those that best suit your individual needs. Ask your doctor for recommendations if any of these products are advised for you.

FINDING THE PRODUCTS YOU NEED

Depending on what they are, incontinence products can be purchased in a number of ways:

- At your local drug store
- At some supermarkets, department; and variety stores
- At surgical supply stores
- From distributors, by mail or phone, often through a catalog
- Directly from the manufacturers
- On the Internet

Some healthcare professionals are not aware of the wide variety of available products and may not feel qualified to give you specific recommendations. In such cases, you can seek out information on your own. One of the easiest ways is on the Internet, where a search under the headings "incontinence" or "urinary incontinence" will yield a long list of sources, including product information. Remember to be cautious about anything you find here, since it is largely unregulated information. It is strongly recommended that you bring this information to your doctor and confirm your findings before making any purchases, unless you are already familiar with the products you want to order.

You can also ask for product recommendations from members of your support group or other people you know who have bladder control problems. The best informed recommendations often come from women who have been using these products for a long time and have tried many different types.

Staff members at medical supply stores can also tell you which products sell well and seem to do the best job for their regular customers. Remember that just because a product is popular, it may not necessarily be the best one for your specific needs.

Another recommended source for learning about currently available products is the *Resource Guide,* published and distributed by the National Association for Continence (see Appendix A). This publication provides basic information about incontinence, a comprehensive list of products, and details on how to contact manufacturers and distributors to obtain these products. The guide also includes advertisements from manufacturers of various incontinence products.

As with many other types of products, incontinence products do not work the same way for everyone. Sometimes it is necessary for you to try different brands or styles before finding one that works well for you. In most cases, your doctor or other healthcare provider will be able to advise and help you with this process.

Be aware that you may not always receive satisfactory help by using just one product. Sometimes you will have to combine two or more products with your treatments in order to achieve the best results. For example, absorbent pads are often used in combination with medication and/or pelvic floor exercise.

Some of these products are available over the counter, but others can only be purchased with your physician's prescription.

How to Select the Right Products

When you look at all the available items, there are certain features you may want to consider as you make your choice about which ones to try.

- *Absorbency:* How much urine can the absorbent product hold before it leaks? How often must it be changed?
- *Disposable or reusable:* Is the product disposable or can it be reused? Which type do you prefer? This is highly individual. For example, you may want a disposable during the day and a reusable product during the night.
- *Cost:* If the product is disposable, will the cost be much higher than the reusable type? If so, which do you prefer?
- *Bulkiness:* Does the product's size cause it to bulge noticeably under your regular clothing? If so, does that bother you? Is there another similar product that is not as bulky and noticeable?

- *Comfort:* Does the product feel comfortable when you wear it and are you usually not aware that you have it on?
- *Portability:* Is it easy to carry the product with you, for example to work or on a trip?
- *Dryness:* Does the product keep your body dry or does it cause problems with your skin due to urine leaking out?
- *Availability:* Is it easy to get the product when you need it?
- *Insurance coverage:* Does your insurance plan pay for the products you want? They can be very costly if used over a long period of time. If they are not covered, are there any substitute products that may be covered? If not, you could ask your physician to help you make an appeal to your insurance company.

Below are descriptions of some of the more popular products for women.

Absorbent Products

The most common way women deal with urinary leakage is by using absorbent products, such as pantiliners, pads, adult diapers, and protective mattress pads. If you decide to use absorbent products to take care of your urinary leakage because you have only an occasional or minimal loss of urine, they may work well and you will be able to continue with your daily life while those around you are not aware of your condition. All absorbent pads are waterproof on the exterior. They may be contoured or rectangular in shape.

Disposable absorbent products are designed to reduce wetness, which can be the cause of many types of skin problems associated with incontinence. Some pads have an ingredient in their material that turns to a gel when wet, providing you with additional protection against leakage and also keeping moisture away from your body.

Many also prevent or minimize odor with different types of built-in deodorants. This feature will make you feel more confident and not so worried about others being aware of your condition.

You may be surprised at the wide variety of absorbent products. For example, one NAFC (National Association for Continence) catalog lists fifty-three different types of liners. These are pads designed for use with regular or waterproof underpants, mostly for women with mild to moderate leakage. You will recognize the heavily publicized brand names Compose and Serenity, but there are many other brands. Find the one that works best for your needs.

There are also reusable absorbent products, such as washable cloth adult diapers, which some women prefer because of greater comfort and lower cost.

Absorbent products are also used in combination with other treatments to catch any possible leaks. Depending on your condition and personal preferences, you can choose from a wide variety of these products, which do not require a prescription.

Light pads, pantiliners, and inserts are thin pads, like the ones used for light menstrual flow, that attach to underwear with an adhesive strip or fit into waterproof garments. They are recommended if you lose only a small amount of urine, usually as a result of stress incontinence, and remain dry at night.

Light to moderate pads attach to your underwear with an adhesive strip or fit into waterproof garments. Designed for light to moderate leakage, which can be due to stress incontinence or urge incontinence, these pads are a good choice if you usually remain dry at night.

Moderate pads, like the ones used for regular menstrual flow, are for the moderate loss of urine due to stress incontinence or urge incontinence. They are recommended if you do not leak a lot of urine at one time, but leak frequently. They include guards, which are slightly heavier and longer than light pads and are used for moderate incontinence. They attach to your underwear with adhesive strips. In addition, there are beltless undergarments, also used for moderate incontinence. Beltless undergarments are also called inserts or liners and can either fit into waterproof underpants or attach to close-fitting regular underpants.

Heavy pads, like the ones used heavy menstrual flow, are best if you have heavy leakage and/or frequent or continuous leakage of urine.

Adult Diapers

Larger, thicker, and more costly than pads, adult diapers can be either disposable or reusable. They are designed to soak up and camouflage leaking urine. The disposable product is made with waterproof plastic on the outside and tabs on the sides to hold them in place. These adult diapers come with or without elastic legs and are available in regular and contoured shapes.

Disposable adult diapers are usually quite bulky and because of the plastic covering, they can also rustle and be somewhat noisy, so if you need them, you will probably want to reserve them for night-time use, if possible. Because they are bulky, it may also be a problem for you to carry a supply with you. Also, they can not be flushed, so disposing of them can be a problem when you are not at home.

Reusable adult diapers are made of cotton and can be washed, just like baby diapers. It is even possible to send them out to a diaper service if desired. Reusable adult diapers are worn with waterproof underpants. They can also be bulky. With this type, carrying a supply and wrapping the used diaper for later washing could also present problems if you are away from home. Some contain special gels to control odor, and all have plastic exteriors to prevent leakage onto clothing.

Both types of adult diapers work best for moderate to heavy incontinence.

Undergarments

Undergarments is the term used for a type of waterproof underwear that is held around your waist with a strap or elastic band. These garments hold absorbent pads in place and provide an added measure of safety over regular underpants in preventing urine from leaking out through the pad. They are used for moderate incontinence.

Protective Underpants or Briefs

Used for moderate to heavy incontinence, these underpants are one-piece garments with waterproof barriers that are pulled up. They are shaped like regular underpants and prevent urinary leakage from absorbent pads. They come in both disposable and reusable types.

Mattress Pads

It is possible that you experience urinary leakage only at night. Or perhaps you leak at different times, including the night. Or you may leak the largest amounts during the night. If any of these apply to you, you will probably want to obtain waterproof protection for your mattress.

Mattress pads with waterproof backing are placed on the mattress to protect it from urinary leakage during the night. They are made by more than forty different companies, come in a variety of sizes and absorbencies, and are recommended if you have moderate to heavy incontinence and leak urine during the night. They are available in both disposable and reusable types.

SKIN CARE PRODUCTS

One side effect of urinary leakage can be problem skin. It is not always possible to clean leaking urine off your skin immediately and soaps can also be very drying. In order to prevent dryness, rashes, and odor, you can use specially formulated cleansers, creams, moisturizers, barrier ointments, skin protectants, and powders that have been designed for problems associated with urinary leakage. There is a wide variety of these types of products, made by many different companies. Be aware that these products are meant not only to deal with skin problems once they develop, but are also for preventive use to protect your skin from any damage that leaking urine may cause.

Deodorizing Products

Sometimes, the urinary leakage odors are made worse because the leaking urine is very concentrated. That can happen when you restrict your fluid intake, trying not to drink too much. There are a number of products to deal with this problem, including deodorizing sprays and wipes, deodorizing drops for neutralizing or masking offensive odors, and tablets that are swallowed and often contain chlorophyllin copper complex to control odors.

INCONTINENCE DEVICES

As part of your treatment, your doctor may recommend a prescription device to help prevent urinary leakage, either for temporary or long-term use. In some cases, there may be several devices to choose from and products can be frequently improved or replaced. When using these devices, it is important to work closely with your doctor to find the ones that work best for you. All the insertion products described below require a doctor's prescription.

SUPPORTIVE DEVICES

If you have stress incontinence, there are supportive or occlusive devices are designed to prevent the leakage of urine. They work either by providing support for the bladder, bladder neck, or urethra; or creating a seal over the end of the urethra which prevents the leakage of urine. However, these devices do not work for urge incontinence. All the studies done on these devices have been with women suffering from only stress incontinence, or mixed incontinence.

• Pessaries: A pessary is a device similar to a diaphragm in design, but heavier. It may be shaped like a ring or a doughnut and comes in a multitude of types. It is inserted in the vagina to reposition a prolapsed organ, such as the bladder or uterus, and keep it in its proper place. The pessary's pressure also helps support the pelvic floor muscles. The pessary does not repair a prolapse, but it can provide relief of the symptoms by repositioning the prolapse.

If you have stress incontinence with some degree of prolapse, cystourethroceles (prolapse of the urethra and bladder) or other similar conditions, a pessary may help you.   You may be able to insert and remove the pessary on your own, but if not, you will need your doctor's assistance. This device should be replaced every one to three months and may be an option if you are unwilling or unable to undergo surgery. Pessaries are available only by prescription and have to be fitted by a physician.

As with any other internal device, pessaries do pose a risk of infection, so if you have one, you should watch for any discharges or unpleasant odors coming from your vagina.

In addition, if you are sexually active, you may find that in order to be comfortable during sexual intercourse, you have to remove the pessary.

The Introl Bladder Neck Support Prosthesis

This is a type of pessary, a specialized device that is inserted into the vagina and used for incontinence associated with bladder or urethral prolapse. The Introl consists of a ring pessary with two prongs coming out of its surface. The two prongs help to restore the bladder neck to its correct anatomical position. The prosthesis can be left in place when you urinate, but it must be removed in order for you to clean it. The manufacturer recommends removing and cleaning it each night before you go to bed and re-inserting it in the morning. The reason they recommend leaving it out for this time period is that continual wearing of the device can cause erosion of the vaginal skin (pressure necrosis) and infection. The device is rather expensive (about $400), and must be properly sized by an experienced professional.

Urethral Inserts

Much smaller than tampons, urethral inserts act as plugs to prevent the leakage of urine. These devices are inserted with an applicator directly into the urethra and when they are in place, they work by blocking the flow of urine into the urethra, preventing unwanted leakage. They are available only by prescription.

You should be aware that there have been some problems reported with the use of these types of devices, including urinary tract infections, especially during the first month of use. Other problems with urethral inserts include pain, discomfort, risk of skin breakdown, and the general reluctance many women have to inserting these devices into their urethras.

RELIANCE URETHRAL INSERT

This brand of urethral insert has a small balloon on the tip that is inflated after proper insertion into the urethra. The balloon holds the insert in place and acts as a plug to prevent urinary leakage. There is a string on the end of the device that hangs outside the body. When you want to urinate, you pull the string to deflate the balloon and remove the device. After urinating, you insert a new one. This device is available only by prescription. [Note: This device has recently been taken off the market, but may be reintroduced at a later date.]

THE FEMSOFT INSERT

Also a disposable urethral insert, the FemSoft is a narrow silicone tube that is covered with a soft, thin silicone sleeve and filled with mineral oil. It has a disposable applicator and is inserted much like a tampon, except that it is placed into the urethra. When properly inserted, the FemSoft cannot be felt. This insert works by preventing urine from leaking out at unwanted times by creating a seal at the neck of the bladder. When you want to urinate, you remove the insert and discard it. Following urination, you insert a new one. This prescription device comes in several different sizes and must be fitted by a doctor.

OCCLUSIVE DEVICES

Occlusive devices are designed to prevent urinary leakage for stress incontinence. They do this by creating a seal over the end of the urethra, thereby preventing the urine from leaking out. There are several different types of occlusive devices, available only with a doctor's prescription.

One of the central problems with occlusive devices, aside from the issues of comfort, skin breakdown, and effectiveness, is that of adhesiveness. Unfortunately, many active people have trouble maintaining a good seal over the urethral opening. The reason is that the device falls off during physical activity, resulting in the sudden occurrence of urinary leakage at potentially very embarrassing times, such as during sports or exercise.

Although urethral inserts and occlusive devices can be very effective in preventing urinary leakage, they are also costly, since they must be replaced often. In some cases, they have to be replaced after each urination. On the other hand, they are not much different in overall cost from absorbent products, such as pads or diapers. Once again, they are a choice you will make depending on your individual condition and your own personal preferences and experiences using them.

Cap Sure and FemAssist Continence Shields

Shaped like suction cups, these occlusive devices are small, round, soft, and made from silicone. They come with a tube of gel, which is used to coat the device prior to insertion over the urethra to cover the urethral opening. Their purpose is to create a suction seal that will prevent any urine from leaking out of the urethral opening. This vacuum seal also holds this device in its proper position over the urethral opening. When you want to urinate, you simply remove the device and urinate normally. You then clean it and replace it over the urethral opening. You can use these devices for about seven days before you have to discard them and replace them with new ones.

THE MINIGUARD PATCH

A disposable foam pad somewhat larger than a postage stamp, the Miniguard is designed to be used only once. On one side, the patch is covered with a gel-like adhesive that holds it in place around the opening of the urethra. When it is positioned properly, it prevents leakage of urine. When you want to urinate, you remove the patch; afterward, you replace it with a new one. Because it is so small, many women prefer this patch to larger, bulkier pads.

Catheters and Self-Catheterization

A catheter is a small, thin tube designed to drain urine from the bladder. There are two types of catheters. One type is placed partially inside the body and left there, in which case it must be changed every few weeks. These indwelling catheters are called Foley catheters.

If you have severe problems, or are not able to visit the bathroom as often as you need to, an indwelling or permanent Foley catheter is an option. It consists of a two-channeled tube with a small balloon at the tip which, when inflated, holds the catheter in place within the bladder. The other, open channel allows urine to drain out of the bladder continuously. A bag attached to your leg receives the drained urine. The bag can be emptied when it is convenient.

The other type of catheter is not permanent, but is used periodically to drain urine by inserting it and removing it from the bladder several times a day. The process of inserting and removing the catheter is called self-intermittent catheterization (SIC). Catheters are generally used for overflow incontinence or incontinence due to neurological problems.

Self-catheterization is often used when a person is unable to urinate properly or completely and a quantity of urine remains after using the toilet, as with overflow incontinence. It is also used if a disease or injury prevents complete natural emptying of the bladder, or for temporary problems of urination while recovering from certain types of surgery. Once mastered, self-catheterization is quick and painless.

In order to do self-catheterization, you sit on the toilet and attempt to urinate normally. You should give yourself sufficient time to empty your bladder as much as you are able, without forcing. Then, you perform the self-catheterization procedure, threading the catheter through your urethra into your bladder. Once the catheter enters your bladder, urine drains out. Once the urine stops draining, you remove the catheter. This procedure is usually performed four to five times per day.

Catheters are made by more than twenty different manufacturers and are available in a variety of materials and styles. In most cases, they can be cleaned and used again. Both types are available only by prescription and require medical instruction and supervision from your doctor or other healthcare professional.

If you have an indwelling Foley catheter either on a temporary or a long-term basis, related products for use with these catheters are also available, including urinary bags, straps, and catheter tube holders.

PART FOUR:
GETTING BETTER

16

COPING WITH THE
EMOTIONAL ISSUES

It is very important not to neglect all the things you can do on your own to improve your health. Sometimes you can prevent incontinence from ever developing in the first place. At other times, you can dramatically improve your condition and occasionally, even cure yourself. You just have to know how. That's where self-help enters the picture.

You really can take charge of your problem and learn to control or sometimes overcome it. The first step of your self-help program is usually a consultation with a doctor who is familiar with incontinence. It is an added benefit if the physician you choose is also familiar with self-help techniques and supports your using them.

These techniques are beneficial because they are:

- Non-invasive
- Inexpensive
- Without side effects
- Low or no risk
- Easily combined with other therapies
- Available to everyone
- Emotionally beneficial (since they actively involve you in your treatment)
- Indicative of your progress.

When you know that you are actively participating in health care and making a positive contribution to getting better, both your physical and emotional outlooks will change for the better.

KEEP YOUR URINARY SYSTEM IN PROPER WORKING ORDER

Whether you are in your teens or twenties, or more mature, there are many things you can do to help keep your urinary system in proper working order.

- Don't smoke; it causes chronic coughing and can also irritate your bladder.
- Consume little or no alcohol; it causes your body to produce a lot of urine in a short period of time.
- Consume little or no caffeine (including coffee, tea, chocolate, and many sodas); it can be a bladder irritant. Caffeine also acts like a diuretic.
- Consume limited sugar and sugar substitutes (aspartame and saccharin), which can be bladder stimulants that irritate the urinary tract, causing urinary urgency or aggravating other existing bladder problems.
- Eat plenty of fiber (including lots of fruit, vegetables, and whole

grains) to avoid constipation. The exact amount of fiber required will vary from person to person. You can find your proper intake by consuming enough high-fiber foods to allow you to avoid constipation.

- Have a liquid intake of at least four to six eight-ounce glasses a day (water, juice, and other non-caffeinated beverages); dehydration can produce concentrated urine that irritates your bladder and can make it overactive.
- Avoid drinking liquids after dinner to prevent bedwetting.
- Avoid drinking excessive liquids; they can aggravate existing incontinence.
- Engage in regular exercise.
- Practice regular pelvic floor exercises, or Kegels.
- Keep to your recommended weight and avoid obesity.
- Only use medications that may cause incontinence when medically necessary (including diuretics, antihistamines, sedatives, antipsychotics, calcium channel blockers).
- Give yourself sufficient time to empty your bladder completely; never rush to leave the bathroom.
- Urinate after sex to avoid bacterial invasions that could lead to urinary tract infections.
- Avoid toilet paper with dyes and perfumes, as well as vaginal deodorants, bath additives; and soaps that have artificial colors and scents. These products can irritate your vagina and urinary system.
- If you experience any urinary leakage, even if it's the first time and even if it's only a small amount, you should consult your doctor.

Combining Self-Help and Medical Care

If you practice the preventive measures listed above, you will be making an important contribution to the maintenance, health, and strength of your urinary system. If all goes well, you may never develop a problem with incontinence. But if you do, it is really important to have a medical evaluation right away. Don't forget that even mild or occasional incontinence can be a symptom of an underlying condition requiring immediate treatment.

Usually, the most effective treatment for urinary incontinence is a combination of self-help techniques and medical intervention specifically designed for your unique case. While you may benefit from only doing regular Kegel exercises, someone else may benefit from Kegels along with biofeedback and some medication.

There are many different combinations of available therapies that can be put together, and the best program for you is the one that you work out on an individual basis with your physician.

If you have a single-minded dedication to helping yourself overcome incontinence, your efforts are certain to yield positive results. While you may not be completely cured, you should be able to successfully manage your condition and in almost all cases, you will be able to carry out all the normal activities of your day-to-day life.

Dealing with Emotional Issues

In Chapter Six, you learned about some of the emotional problems that you may have to deal with. Even if your condition is very mild, you may still feel embarrassed, fearful, anxious, angry, ashamed, depressed, or generally negative about yourself and your life. These unpleasant emotions are even more likely if you don't seek medical help and feel compelled to hide your problem.

The stigma associated with your condition can cause you to suffer needless emotional pain. Some studies show that depression, anxiety, and phobias can be associated with urinary leakage. In fact, in extreme cases, women have said that considering everything they have to deal with, "life is not worth living."

That is sad, considering that there are effective treatments for this condition once it is properly diagnosed. Do not let yourself fall into despair, although it is understandable that you may feel extremely unhappy and discouraged from time to time.

Even if you are aware of effective treatments and decide not to go for help, or if you see a doctor and don't receive the proper diagnosis or treatment, or if you have a severe condition that does not respond well to treatment or takes a long time to improve, you may find yourself feeling depressed. That's why it's so important for you to be aware of your emotions and to make sure not to neglect them. Here's how.

Taking Positive Steps to Cope with Your Condition

If you are having bladder control problems and have not yet seen a physician, you should do so right away. If you have seen a doctor for your condition and have not received satisfactory help, take immediate steps to find another doctor, using the guidelines presented in Chapter Seven.

If you have a condition that has been treated but has not improved as much as you anticipated, discuss it with your physician and find out if there is anything else that can be done, or if you just need to be more patient.

Getting Help from Therapists and Support Groups

As with any chronic problem, you may feel a need for emotional support and want to consider therapy or a community support group (see below). Therapy and support groups can help you with:

- Admitting that you need help with your incontinence problem
- Telling your loved ones about your incontinence
- Taking the first step in finding a doctor to treat your incontinence.
- Dealing with the difficult aspects of the disorder, such as leakage at inconvenient or embarrassing times
- Deciding how to incorporate your condition into your job schedule
- Maintaining a positive attitude while you are in the process of being diagnosed and treated
- Finding the strength to do everything you can to help yourself, such as pelvic floor exercises and other behavioral modification techniques

- Coping with the negative emotions you may experience as a result of your condition
- Becoming more assertive, when necessary, in getting the help you need
- Developing a sense of humor about your problem
- Developing a positive self-image

Therapists

In some cases, a good therapist can be an important part of your course of treatment. Even if you think you have your problem in hand, the psychological effects of battling this disorder can be overwhelming at times. If you have the opportunity to work with a therapist who is familiar with the many problems associated with urinary incontinence, it will definitely help.

Remember, too, that some types of incontinence are caused by emotional triggers. For example, if you are suffering from unusual stress or anxiety, your emotional state can affect your body and result in bladder problems. So your emotions can be the *cause* of incontinence, the *result* of incontinence, and sometimes, both cause and effect. A good therapist can help you sort out your emotions and deal with them more successfully.

Support Groups

You will find it easier to recover if you have the support of others, especially those who have the same condition and really understand what you are experiencing. That is why support groups, made up of people with the same types of problems, can be so helpful.

When should you seek out a support group? The sooner the better, because:

- You will not feel embarrassed discussing incontinence with others who suffer from the same condition.
- People attending support groups generally have an extensive knowledge about this condition.

- You can get physician referrals from support group members.
- You will hear from people who have conditions exactly like yours and learn how they are coping with it.
- You can feel comfortable asking all the questions that are on your mind.
- You will realize how many people have your condition and how many ways there are of successfully coping with it.
- You will meet people you can call when you need information or emotional support.
- You will be able to help others if you continue going to meetings, make every effort to improve your condition, and share your experiences with other group members.

It's a fact that many women are motivated to seek help only when, after years of silent pain, they meet someone else with the same condition, or hear someone talk about it on television or read something about it in the newspaper and discover how much they can do for themselves. That is exactly what can happen at your first support group meeting.

It takes a lot of courage to pick up the phone, find out where a support group is meeting, go there, and walk through the door. But as soon as you do, you will find a warm, welcoming feeling from the other people in the room because every one of them has gone through the same experience.

Do you have to attend a lot of meetings or keep going for months or years? Of course not. You can go once and if you don't feel the meeting is beneficial, you don't have to go back. Or you can try a different group. Or you can go a few times until you feel you have the information you need or decide that you no longer want to attend. Support groups do not involve any kind of obligation and they are usually free, with a small voluntary donation at the end of the meeting.

Finding a Support Group

Although there are many urinary incontinence support groups throughout the country, finding them can often be difficult. Here are some suggestions for locating a support group in your area:

- Ask your doctor or other healthcare provider.
- Call Continence Restored, 203-348-0601 (see Appendix A).
- Contact the gynecology, urology or urogynecology department of your local hospital.
- Ask a friend or relative who has had the same problem.
- Ask the manager of your local medical supplies store.
- Check the telephone book under "incontinence," "continence," "bladder control," or "support groups," and look through the health services section of the government pages for incontinence.

If you are not successful in finding a local support group, you can start one of your own. Continence Restored will give you information and help you to set one up.

Waiting for Treatment Results

There is no hard and fast rule about how long it should take for you to see positive results from any given treatment. There are simply too many variables. Results can depend on:

- The type of incontinence
- The severity of your condition
- How long you have been incontinent
- Your age and physical condition
- The underlying causes and their treatment
- Other medical conditions you may have
- How well you follow your doctor's directions
- Support from your family, friends, and co-workers
- Your patience

Patience

It may sometimes take you a while to find the right doctor, get a proper diagnosis, and treat all the underlying causes of your urinary leakage, but if you are patient, improvements will eventually begin to occur.

Once you have started treatment, you will probably want to ask your doctor how long you will have to wait for results, what all your options are, and if some other treatment will work in case your recommended therapy doesn't have the results you are looking for.

You will also want information about everything you can do on your own to improve your condition. Chances are, you will follow up and do whatever it takes. More than anything, you want to regain control over your bladder and will do whatever is necessary to achieve that result.

Patience is extremely important. Diagnosing and treating incontinence can be a very complex and time-consuming task and it is really important for both you and your physician to persist until you experience some positive results.

Maybe you are not a patient sort of person. Perhaps, even if your condition is severe, you expect to cure it immediately. If that is the case and surgery is an option for you, you may decide to have surgery—not because it is the treatment of last resort, but because it is the treatment most likely to cure you quickly.

On the other hand, you may be a different type of woman, one who wants to avoid surgery at all costs. If that is the case, you may be willing to spend weeks and months doing pelvic floor exercises, going for biofeedback treatments, and taking medication in order to avoid a surgical operation.

If you are fortunate, you may see good results in a few days or a few weeks. Otherwise, you may need a much longer time before your condition begins to improve.

Whatever happens, the important thing is never give up! Set your mind and your heart on conquering this problem and find a way to persist despite any difficulties you may have to face along the way. If you refuse to give up, remain patient, and keep working at finding a solution, you will eventually succeed.

17

FUTURE TREATMENTS

What kinds of treatments for urinary incontinence and its associated problems are on the horizon? Does it look as though some miraculous therapies will soon be available?

Of course, it is everyone's dream that miracle cures will be discovered for all disorders, but it is more realistic to expect that new, improved therapies will soon be available and they will make treatment easier and more effective. Drug companies are always working on new medications, but the process of development and approval is quite expensive and can sometimes take many years. Here are some of the new therapies that may be available in the near future:

- Medications such as newer anticholinergic agents that are more selective (effective) and specific (with fewer side effects) than the ones now on the market. These new drugs will be able to focus better on their urinary targets and be more effective in doing their jobs in helping to treat urinary incontinence, while avoiding unpleasant side effects.

• The use of medications or drugs applied directly into your bladder that decrease sensory input (such as capsaicin) could be very useful in the treatment of urge incontinence.

• A better, more stable and suitable tissue substitute for use in bladder augmentation surgery or sling surgery may be developed through biotechnology and tissue-engineering techniques.

• Gene therapy or the possibility of directly inserting tiny amounts of DNA and other genetic material into individual cells in damaged urinary organs may repair them and allow them to function better.

In the mean time, you should remember that there are many effective ways to treat urinary incontinence today. If you have a problem, even a little one, it's really time to see your doctor and take care of it. Join the millions of women who have found help. It's there, waiting for you, right now. Go to it!

Appendix A:

ORGANIZATIONS

There are many organizations that provide information and help for women with bladder control problems. It is not possible to include them all here, so we have selected a few that have proven useful for many women. You can telephone, write, or e-mail these organizations to request printed information on various aspects of bladder control problems and assistance with finding a qualified doctor.

There are so many companies that manufacture and sell incontinence products, it is not possible to list them here. These companies often provide printed material about their products and about incontinence. See Chapter Fifteen for information on how to find them.

THE NATIONAL ASSOCIATION
FOR CONTINENCE (NAFC)

Toll-free phone: 1-800-BLADDER (1-800-252-3337)
Telephone: 864-579-7900
Fax: 864-579-7902
Address: P. O. Box 8310, Spartanburg, SC 29305-8310
Internet: www.nafc.org

NAFC is a nonprofit organization that was formerly known as HIP (Help for Incontinent People) and is one of the best resources for help and information on women's incontinence. According to their mission statement, "NAFC's purpose is to be the leading source of education, advocacy, and support to the public and to the health professional about the causes, prevention, diagnosis, treatments, and management alternatives for incontinence."

Founded in 1982, NAFC publishes a quarterly newsletter, *Quality Care*, which is sent to members. They distribute a comprehensive directory, *The Resource Guide-Products and Services for Incontinence*, which has over 100 pages listing more than 1,000 products. They also provide a starter kit for those who want to begin a support group and distribute NAFC Fact Sheets (informational brochures), books, and audiovisual materials to educate the public and healthcare professionals about incontinence. NAFC also has a Continence Resource Service (CRS), a database of doctors, to help members and non-members find qualified doctors in their area.

THE SIMON FOUNDATION FOR CONTINENCE

Toll-free telephone: 1-800-23-SIMON (1-800-237-4666)
Telephone: 847-864-3913
Fax: 847-864-9758
Address: P. O. Box 835, Wilmette IL 60091
Internet: www.simonfoundation.org

A not-for-profit organization, The Simon Foundation's purpose is to educate the public about incontinence and extend help to those with bladder control problems and their families. This organization provides members with a quarterly newsletter, *The Informer,* has online discussions about incontinence on its website; provides article reprints, books, videos, and CDs about incontinence; and supplies information on recent conferences on incontinence.

On request, The Simon Foundation will send you a free information packet, including a list of resources and a sample copy of their newsletter. Founder Cheryle Gartley also provides information to members of the public who write or fax her directly through The Simon Foundation.

AMERICAN UROLOGICAL ASSOCIATION

Toll-free telephone: 1-877-DRY LIFE (1-800-379-5433)
Telephone: 410-727-1100
Fax: 410-223-4370
Internet: www.drylife.org

The American Urological Association provides two types of information to the general public: a copy of their treatment guide for incontinence and a list of physicians in your area who specialize in incontinence. You can also get a physician referral online at their website, as well as read and download a copy of their informational brochure, "You Are Not Alone."

AMERICAN FOUNDATION FOR UROLOGIC DISEASE (AFUD)

Toll-free telephone: 1-877-846-3222
Address: 1128 North Charles Street, Baltimore MD 21201
Internet: www.afud.org

AFUD is a nonprofit organization that works to prevent and cure urologic disease through education of the general public and healthcare professionals, and through supporting increased medical research into urologic diseases. The organization's toll-free number listed above is their "Take Control Hot Line," through which you can request printed information on topics such as the overactive bladder and interstitial cystitis.

NATIONAL INSTITUTE OF DIABETES AND DIGESTIVE AND KIDNEY DISEASES (NIDDK)

Toll-free telephone: 1-800-891-5388
Fax: 301-907-8906
Internet: www.niddk.nih.gov

The NIDDK is a government service of the National Institutes of Health under the United States Department of Health and Human Services. It provides free consumer and doctor kits, including publications such as "Bladder Control for Women," "Your Body's Design for Bladder Control," "Daily Bladder Diary," "Talking to Your Healthcare Team About Bladder Control," "Exercising Your Pelvic Muscles," "Menopause and Bladder Control," "Pregnancy, Childbirth, and Bladder Control," and "Your Medicines and Bladder Control."

Online, NIDDK provides detailed information on incontinence in women, including types of incontinence, diagnosis, and treatment. They will also respond to inquiries for specific information on kidney and urologic diseases through e-mail, fax, and regular mail, and will send you free publications on all aspects of these diseases. In addition, they have an extensive database of health education materials for both lay people and health care professionals, which includes fact sheets, brochures and audiovisual materials.

CONTINENCE RESTORED, INC.

Telephone: 203-348-0601
Address: 407 Strawberry Hill Avenue, Stamford CT 06902

Continence Restored, Inc. is a non-profit organization that provides information about bladder control problems to the general public and to manufacturers of products for bladder control. They also assist in the establishment of support groups and help people find an existing support group in their area. Continence Restored will send you an informational article about urinary incontinence if you send them a request, along with a #10 stamped self-addressed envelope.

NATIONAL BLADDER FOUNDATION

Toll-free telephone: 1-877-BLADDER (1-877-252-3337)
Telephone: 203-431-0005
Fax: 203-431-0008
Address: P. O. Box 1095, Ridgefield CT 06877
Internet: www.bladder.org

The National Bladder Foundation provides information on incontinence, including details on types, causes, diagnosis, and treatment. Its stated mission is "to achieve the rapid discovery of cures and preventive interventions for the most common bladder diseases, through the support of research." The National Bladder Foundation also compiles government statistics on the incidence of bladder conditions, including incontinence, and sponsors symposia throughout the country. You can find detailed information on urinary incontinence and other bladder conditions on their website and can also enter your name and address for their mailing list.

If you telephone, you can talk to someone about your specific bladder problem. The Foundation will also provide information and referrals to other sources relevant to your specific bladder disorder and will send you free brochures dealing with your problem.

THE NATIONAL COUNCIL ON AGING

Toll-free telephone: 1-800-424-9046
Telephone: 202-479-1200
Fax: 202-479-0735
Address: 409 Third Street SW, Washington DC 20024
Internet: www.ncoa.org

Founded in 1950, The National Council on Aging is a private, non-profit association dedicated to promoting the interests of older Americans, including health issues. They provide a publication on over-active bladders entitled "A Patient Guide for Effective Communication with Health Care Professionals," and have extensive information about incontinence online, including sample voiding diaries.

THE AMERICAN ACADEMY
OF MEDICAL ACUPUNCTURE
(IN LOS ANGELES)

Telephone: 213-937-5514
Fax: 213-937-0959
Internet: www.medicalacupuncture.org

They can provide you with a referral to an acupuncturist in your area. Always be certain that the practitioner you choose has proper training and a state license if one is required where you live. You should also find out if the acupuncturist has experience treating urinary incontinence.

Appendix B

BOOKS

The following books are recommended for those who want further information about bladder control problems. They are often available at public libraries and can also be purchased from local bookstores and online booksellers, including amazon.com and barnes&noble.com.

Jerry Blavais, M.D., *Conquering Bladder and Prostate Problems.* New York: Plenum Trade, 1998.

This book has sections on incontinence in women and goes into detail about how the urinary system works and how bladder control problems develop. It is a comprehensive guide offering useful information on different types of incontinence and their treatment.

Kathryn L. Burgio, Ph.D., K. Lynette Pearce, R.N., C.R.N.P., and Angelo J. Lucco, M.D., *Staying Dry*. Baltimore, Maryland: Johns Hopkins University Press, 1989.

This short book provides step-by-step instructions on such practical information as how to do Kegels, how to keep a voiding diary, and how to understand your bladder control problem. It is a helpful introduction to incontinence.

Rebecca Chalker and Kristene E. Whitmore, M.D., *Overcoming Bladder Disorders*, New York: Harper & Row, 1990.

This compassionate guide deals with both the physical and emotional components of bladder problems and provides comprehensive information on every aspect of dealing with them, including finding a doctor, diagnosis and treatment. It does not include the newer treatments, but has much useful information.

Cheryle B. Gartley, *Managing Incontinence*. Ottawa, Illinois: Jameson Books, Inc. , 1985.

Gartley is the founder and president of the Simon Foundation. Her book, written many years ago, still provides an understanding introduction to incontinence and has good material on the psychological impact of this health problem.

Diane Kaschak-Newman, R.N.C., M.S.N., C.R.N.P., F.A.A.N.,*The Urinary Incontinence Sourcebook*. Chicago: Lowell House, 1999.

This reference book is an excellent source for products and services available to women with urinary incontinence. The author is an adult nurse practitioner specializing in the diagnosis and treatment of urinary incontinence.

ABOUT THE AUTHORS

Eric S. Rovner, M.D., is co-director of the Center for Incontinence and Pelvic Floor Disorders at the University of Pennsylvania Medical School, co-director of the videourodynamics unit of the Department of Radiology, assistant professor of surgery in radiology, and a board-certified urologist. He has lectured widely on incontinence in women and has written and co-authored scientific papers for several medical journals, including many on incontinence and related issues.

Dr. Rovner received his undergraduate degree from Johns Hopkins University and his medical degree from the Albert Einstein College of Medicine. He lives with his family in Cherry Hill, New Jersey.

Alan J. Wein, M.D., is professor and chair of the Division of Urology at the University of Pennsylvania School of Medicine, and co-director of the voiding function and dysfuction and urologic oncology programs there.

Dr. Wein has lectured widely on incontinence and is the author or co-author of many scientific articles and urologic textbooks. He serves on the editorial boards of twelve urologic journals. He co-chairs World Health Organization International Consultations on Incontinence.

Dr. Wein received his undergraduate degree from Princeton and his medical degree from the University of Pennsylvania. He lives with his family in Gladwyne, Pennsylvania.

Donna Caruso is a freelance writer who has written and co-authored many books and articles and who specializes in health and medical issues. She lives on Long Island, New York.

INDEX